Rebels with a Cause

of related interest

Psychodrama
A Beginner's Guide
Zoran Djuric, Jasna Veljkovic and Miomir Tomic
ISBN 1 84310 411 3

Sambadrama
The Arena of Brazilian Psychodrama
Edited and translated by Zoltán Figusch
Forewords by Adam Blatner and José Fonseca
ISBN 1 84310 363 X

Communicating with Children and Adolescents
Action for Change
Edited by Anne Bannister and Annie Huntington
ISBN 1 84310 025 8

Drama Workshops for Anger Management and Offending Behaviour
James Thompson
ISBN 1 85302 702 2

Introduction to Dramatherapy
Theatre and Healing – Ariadne's Ball of Thread
Sue Jennings
Foreword by Clare Higgins
ISBN 1 85302 115 6

Rebels with a Cause

Working with Adolescents Using Action Techniques

Mario Cossa

Foreword by Zerka Moreno

Jessica Kingsley Publishers
London and Philadelphia

Appendices A, B, and C (marked ✓) may be photocopied for personal use
without permission from the publisher.

First published in 2006
by Jessica Kingsley Publishers
116 Pentonville Road
London N1 9JB, UK
and
400 Market Street, Suite 400
Philadelphia, PA 19106, USA

www.jkp.com

Library of Congress Cataloging in Publication Data

Cossa, Mario.
    Rebels with a cause : working with adolescents using action techniques / Mario Cossa ; foreword by Zerka
Moreno.-- 1st American pbk. ed.
        p. cm.
    Includes bibliographical references and index.
    ISBN-13: 978-1-84310-379-0 (pbk. : alk. paper)
    ISBN-10: 1-84310-379-6 (pbk. : alk. paper) 1. Drama--Therapeutic use. 2. Group psychotherapy for
teenagers. 3. Group psychotherapy for youth. I. Title.
    RJ505.P89C67 2006
    616.89'1523--dc22

                                    2005018681

British Library Cataloguing in Publication Data
A CIP catalogue record for this book is available from the British Library

ISBN-13: 978 184310 379 0
ISBN-10: 1 84310 379 6

Printed and Bound in Great Britain by
Athenaeum Press, Gateshead, Tyne and Wear

A sacred space is a place where we,
as humans, can be at our very best.
(Zerka Moreno, workshop conversation, May 1992)

For Zerka,
who makes all spaces sacred.

Contents

ACKNOWLEDGEMENTS   11

FOREWORD BY ZERKA MORENO   13

PREFACE   15

INTRODUCTION   17

PART I WARM-UP: PHILOSOPHICAL AND
THEORETICAL BASIS   **19**

1   Adolescents in Action   21
     Why adolescents? A unique therapeutic opportunity   21
     Defining key terms   22
     Why use action methods with adolescent groups?   24
     Moreno's universalia of psychotherapy   26
     Summary   33

2   Viewing Adolescence from a Developmental Perspective   35
     Stages and phases of group development   36
     The developmental tasks of adolescence   41
     The developmental continuum of adolescence   43
     Summary   51

3   The Therapeutic Spiral™ as a Framework for Working
     with Adolescent Groups   53
     Roles of restoration: connecting to strengths   54
     Roles of observation: engaging and disengaging appropriately 57
     Roles of containment: dealing with affect productively   58
     Summary   61

4   Leadership and Group Norms   63
     The role of the leader(s)   63
     The importance of group norms   66
     Summary   73

PART II ACTION: UTILIZING ACTION TECHNIQUES AT VARIOUS STAGES OF GROUP DEVELOPMENT   75

5   Action Techniques for the Beginning Stage   77
   Initial contact with group members   77
   Introductory group sessions   81
   Developing the beginning stage   85
   Summary   90

6   Action Techniques for the Transition Stage   91
   Getting unstuck   91
   Moving forward   97
   Summary   99

7   Action Techniques for the Working Group   101
   Building personal, interpersonal, and transpersonal strengths   102
   Developing the ability to observe from within and without   105
   Developing strategies for containment of intense affect   108
   Working with life issues in action   112
   Summary   120

8   Action Techniques for Termination   123
   Awareness of ending at the group's beginning   124
   Rehearsals for ending   125
   Terminating the group   130
   Summary   133

PART III SHARING: OTHER APPLICATIONS OF ACTION TECHNIQUES AND CONSIDERATIONS FOR THEIR IMPLEMENTATION   135

9   Adapting Action Techniques to the Population and Setting   137
   Working with special populations   138
   Working in special settings and situations   152
   Summary   158

10   Practical Considerations for Developing
     and Implementing Adolescent Action Groups   159
     Importance of integrating theory and philosophy with practice   159
     Fitting strategies to actual needs of group or population   162
     Summary   167

APPENDIX A: SAMPLE INFORMATION PACK FOR PARTICIPANTS
              AND FAMILIES   169

APPENDIX B: SAMPLE INTAKE AND PERMISSION FORMS   173

APPENDIX C: SAMPLE GROUP NORMS   177

APPENDIX D: OTHER IDEAS FOR OPENING AND CLOSING CIRCLES,
              WARM-UPS, COOL-DOWNS, AND DE-ROLING   181

REFERENCES   197

SUBJECT INDEX   199

AUTHOR INDEX   207

Acknowledgements

First and foremost, I acknowledge my dear friend and colleague of many years, Sally Ember, Ed.D., for her incredible contribution to my overall professional development as well as to this book. Sally has been a source of inspiration, a sounding board, and an engaged cohort on countless projects. She has served as front-line copy editor and proofreader for this book (as well as for other recently published material) and has helped me clarify ideas, organize information, and develop my skill as a writer. She has also tried to teach me to use a comma consistently and correctly (you cannot win them all). Without her, this manuscript would never have reached the publication stage.

I also acknowledge and appreciate the many young people I have worked with over the years in many capacities. They have enriched my life with their enthusiasm, passion, struggles, and achievements. They have been my greatest teachers and guides. This is especially true of those youth who were part of ACTINGOUT, a program I developed and directed from 1989 to 2003.

I acknowledge as well my teachers, mentors, and supervisors during my training as a psychodramatist and in developing the ACTINGOUT program. They have inspired me to learn, encouraged me to grow, and stimulated me to delve more deeply. Among them are: Michael Conforti, Lindsay Freeze, Jonathan Fox, Kate Hudgins, Carol Jue, Penny Lewis, Sharon Mangan, Jacala Mills, Zerka Moreno, Joe Schapiro, Guy Taylor, and Francis Warman.

Special thanks to my "international family" in the USA (especially Barbara, Sandra, Marty, and Stephen), England (especially Chip and Enid), South Africa (especially Vivyan and Jacinda), New Zealand (especially Marlyn, Martin, and Selina), and Australia (especially Penny, Linda, Kaya, Martin, Ailis, and Ella) who have allowed me to travel the world and always feel at home. I have a fond appreciation for Australia, within whose borders most of this book was written.

Finally, I would like to acknowledge the staff of the ACTINGOUT program, especially my colleague and co-worker for many years, Kamala Burden, as well as the many fine graduate interns from Antioch/New England Graduate School who served the program. At the same time, I acknowledge the collegial staff working at ACTINGOUT's sponsoring organization, Monadnock Family Services, a community mental health agency in Keene, New Hampshire (USA). All were instrumental in the development of ACTINGOUT as an idea as well as a program. Several drafts of Part I of this book were completed while I was on sabbatical from the program/agency during the winter of 2000–2001.

Appendices A, B, and C, which offer sample forms for organizing a group program, are taken from material developed at ACTINGOUT.

Foreword

In this book, Mario Cossa has undertaken a selected approach to working with youngsters on the edge. As a certified trainer, educator, and practitioner in psychodrama and group psychotherapy in the mold of J.L. Moreno, Mario has managed to bring together his philosophy, theory and methods in a superb book.

The idea that children and young folk are merely small adults has existed in our western cultures for centuries. It is only fairly recently that it became clear that they needed and deserved a special kind of attention. Psychotherapeutic approaches for working with youth are also of comparatively recent date and require an entirely different process from working with adults.

Of even more recent date are the findings by researchers in neurology who have studied the MRIs taken in youth from 12 years of age up until 25. These researchers have discovered and reported that the prefrontal lobe of the adolescent brain, the site where judgment is found, does not fully develop until the mid-20s.

It is small wonder that we see such evidence daily of struggles with issues of judgment in youth as well as many behavioral difficulties. We used to think that the hormones and their upheaval were partly the reason. Now we have evidence that the combination of physical, hormonal, and neurological changes makes matters far more complex as youth negotiate an increasingly complex world.

Mario Cossa has produced a very fine and complete guide to using action methods effectively and appropriately with adolescent groups. His book opens up new vistas and is a fine guide into this area of work, to which he has been devoted for a long time. It deserves serious appreciation, not only by professional persons, but also by the general reader. It is a cornerstone in the field of psychotherapy as well as a book for anyone who is concerned with the welfare of our younger generation.

Zerka Moreno
The Moreno Institute

Preface

I approached the writing of this book with profound respect and appreciation for the many adolescents with whom I have worked over time and in many capacities. The title, *Rebels with a Cause*, reflects both my perspective on the meaning and purpose of the adolescent experience as well as a cinematic influence on my personal history.

I was a teen myself when I first saw the film *Rebel without a Cause*. I identified with the issues, frustrations, and confusion of the characters played by James Dean, Sal Mineo, and Natalie Wood. Years later, I found myself working with youth who were grappling with these same issues, dressed in the clothing of a newer generation. As my understanding of and appreciation for the adolescent experience grew, I began to see that there really is a "cause" for rebellion, for pushing against the established order. It is an integral part of the growth experience. In 1995, I first used the title, in my rearranged form, for a workshop I co-presented at a conference of the American Society for Group Psychotherapy and Psychodrama (ASGPP).

I remember a "humorous" essay I once read that proposed that adolescence be considered a mental disorder and assigned a place in the *Diagnostic and Statistical Manual* of the day. Although this essay appeared funny at first, I later saw it as an illustration of an attitude that impedes meaningful communication between many adults and the youth they endeavor to serve. In contrast, my view of adolescence and of adolescents is a celebratory one, which I hope to share with you in this book.

Mario Cossa
Melbourne, Australia, 2005

Introduction

I began working with adolescents in the early 1970s, when I was barely past my own adolescence. I was an advisor to a high school ecology club and was often stopped by teachers asking for my own hall pass as I made my way to meet with my group. It has been many years since that type of mistake has been made.

In the following years I worked as a junior high school science teacher and as a theatre arts instructor. It was in this last capacity that the seeds of my current career were planted. In the early 1980s, I worked with an organization called the Children's Performing Arts Center (CPAC), offering programs for teens, as well as doing educational programs in the schools, using theatre to explore various curricular areas.

In 1984, a parents' group from a local high school approached CPAC to develop a program about substance abuse. Working with a local therapist and a group of high school students, we created a show entitled "Sex, Drugs, and Rock & Roll." Through this process, and subsequent groups with teens, I began to see the way in which the work I was doing was as much about supporting youth in exploring their own issues as it was about creating educational theatre.

Soon after, I began working as a case manager for a nonprofit organization, Youth Services, Inc. (YSI), whose mission was to work with court-adjudicated youth and their families. I also enrolled in the Antioch/New England Graduate School program in counseling psychology, with an interest in therapeutic theatre. I had heard of psychodrama and had a vague notion of drama therapy, and I wanted to know more.

During my first matriculated year at Antioch, I was a home-based, family therapist for YSI, which also served as my graduate internship. During my second year, I was planning to concentrate my studies in the areas of group and expressive therapies and to begin independent training in psychodrama. I needed a significantly new internship, since this was a requirement of the program.

One morning at a YSI staff meeting, our director opened by asking, "Where is your passion?" He explained that the board of the agency wanted us to develop new programs for youth to help *prevent* court involvement. It was his belief that, out of our passions, we would design good programs. "I have an idea," I said, and the rest, as they say, is history.

In September 1989, the ACTINGOUT™ (AO) program accepted its first members. The program combined expressive arts group therapy with training and performance opportunities in issue-oriented, audience-interactive, improvisational theatre. During the 14 years in which I served as program director, AO moved several times (changing sponsors, or "umbrella" agencies), and is now (2005) a key member of the Consortium of Alternative and Prevention Programs of Monadnock Family Services, a community mental health agency serving southwestern New Hampshire.

In 1996, we published *ACTING OUT: The Workbook – A Guide to the Development and Presentation of Issue-oriented, Audience-interactive, Improvisational Theatre* (Cossa *et al.* 1996), which focused on our theatre education work. Friends then encouraged me to write another book about the clinical work we were doing.

After five years of thinking about the structure and content, but with little time to actually put words on paper, I took a three-month sabbatical from AO. During this time, finally, I began to commit the thoughts and experiences of many years into the form you now hold. In July 2003, I took my leave of ACTINGOUT to travel and train others around the world, and to finish this book. Although I no longer work for ACTINGOUT, its history, up until I left, was my history as well, and my experiences there serve as source material for much of this book.

No book can be a definitive work on a subject that keeps evolving. Our operational understanding of therapeutic theory and practice is "of the moment," but we should not hold on to it too tightly. Rather, as we do with the youth we serve, we contain the moment with open hands, providing the support necessary for it to develop in its own way and time, and allow our understanding to grow along with it.

For information on my forthcoming workshops and events, as well as details of my other publications, please visit my website at http://pws.prserv.net/dramario/

Part I

Warm-up: Philosophical and Theoretical Basis

Chapter 1 lays a foundation for this book by exploring the unique therapeutic opportunity available at adolescence, and the reasons that action techniques are particularly suited to adolescent groups. It also provides definitions of key terms. This chapter then goes on to examine the uniqueness of the adolescent experience in terms of Moreno and Moreno's (1975) *universalia of psychotherapy* and how they apply to working with adolescent populations. These universalia are at the core of the philosophical framework of this book and provide a view of the adolescent experience that is both respectful and practical.

Chapter 2 views adolescence from a developmental perspective. It first compares parallels between individual development and the development of a group, and then notes the differing challenges at each stage of group development. It also addresses the particular developmental needs of adolescents, and the ways that action strategies are particularly suited to supporting the meeting of those needs in group work.

Chapter 3 provides an overview of the ways in which elements from the Therapeutic Spiral Model™ (Hudgins 2002) for the utilization of psychodrama with survivors of trauma can act as a framework for further refining developmental goals for an adolescent group.

Chapter 4 explores principles of effective group leadership. It also examines the benefits of establishing and adhering to reliable group norms in addressing the needs of the group and its member.

CHAPTER I

Adolescents in Action

In the opening paragraph of a journal article about adolescents, drama therapist, Renée Emunah (1990) wrote: "Most people steer away from them. They are considered hostile, moody, narcissistic, withdrawn, aggressive, rebellious, and unpredictable....Therapists seem to be either particularly reluctant or particularly drawn to working with them" (p.101). As a therapist, I fall into the second category. The challenges, wonders, and rewards of working with adolescents have remained, for me, motivating forces in my work and in my ongoing desire to focus a major portion of my life's professional endeavors on this population.

Why adolescents? A unique therapeutic opportunity

During adolescence, there is a unique opportunity for therapeutic intervention that exists at no other time in the life cycle. As young people move into this period of their lives, they revisit the developmental challenges of childhood, with the peer group assuming a role of support and influence parallel to that held by the family during childhood. With appropriate support from caring adults and connection to a positive peer group, the earlier challenges that have been met can be revisited at a new level of awareness. Additionally, those challenges that have not been successfully negotiated can be revisited and appropriate repairs made. Whether their previous experience was positive or dysfunctional, this revisiting of earlier challenges provides experience that supports young people to face the challenges of their current developmental stage more fully resourced.

Given the primary role that peers play at this time of life, working with adolescents in groups optimizes these interpersonal connections, and provides a kind of support and safety that adults alone, no matter how well intentioned, cannot provide. Adolescents are testing the safety of the adult world, and need the support of thoughtful and caring adults, as well as peer interaction, while they negotiate the difficult transition from child to adult. A positive group experience, in which young people are respected for who they are, and are invited to explore, rather than ordered to "behave," can be truly life changing.

Later in this chapter, I explore reasons for utilizing action methods in working with adolescent groups. First, however, I will define the key terms used throughout this book.

Defining key terms

To avoid confusion or misunderstanding, and realizing that practitioners of action techniques have an idiosyncratic view of the work they do, I offer my understanding of the definitions for the following terms: *action methods, psychodrama and sociodrama, sociometry, drama therapy*, and *adolescence*.

Action methods

Action methods refer to those educational and therapeutic techniques that involve having participants physically involved in activity instead of just talking and listening. For the purposes of this book, I focus primarily on psychodrama (including sociodrama and sociometry) and drama therapy. I am personally indebted to the incredible contribution that dance/movement therapy (DMT) has made to my understanding and practice of the above modalities. However, since it is neither an area of expertise I possess, nor a "language" in which I am fluent, using DMT with adolescents will not be a focus of this work.

Psychodrama and sociodrama

Psychodrama, from its Greek roots, means, literally "the soul in action." With its initial letter capitalized, Psychodrama refers to a body of philosophical, therapeutic, educational, action-based techniques and approaches as first introduced by J.L. Moreno (1964), and further developed by countless practitioners over time. From this perspective, psychodrama (with a lower case "p") and sociodrama are each a part of this field.

I use the term psychodrama to refer to those action techniques in which individuals use enactment to explore material that is identified as specific and personal to them. For example, Sally is exploring *her* relationship with *her* mother, or Marty is exploring the ambivalence *she* feels about moving here from another state.

In those cases in which we are exploring a group issue, or a generic issue common to members of the group, we use the term sociodrama to indicate this particular type of Psychodramatic activity. For example, the group is exploring what it feels like to accept new members into a group that had previously been closed, or the group is exploring the kinds of conflicts that teens often have inter-personally, with parents, or internally, about going to a new school.

Sociometry

Sociometry is the science, created and pioneered by Moreno (1993), which explores and measures the kinds and amounts of interpersonal connections within a group, and the types of choices group members make, based on various criteria. For example, which members of the group are connected to which other members, and which are "isolates"? And to whom do group members turn when they are looking for advice, for support, etc.?

Through sociometric exploration, we can discover how many lines of connec-tion to and from particular individuals in a group currently exist. We can also look at the intensity of these connections, as well as how positive/negative they are. Although not sociometry per se, we also call activities sociometric when they are used either to explore and illuminate for the group the connections that exist, or to build new and positive connections.

Drama therapy

Drama therapy is defined by the National Association for Drama Therapy (2005) as follows:

> Drama therapy is the systematic and intentional use of drama/theatre processes and products to achieve the therapeutic goals of symptom relief, emotional and physical integration, and personal growth. [It] facilitates the client's ability to tell his/her story, solve problems, set goals, express feelings appropriately, achieve catharsis, extend the depth and breadth of inner expe-rience, improve interpersonal skills and relationships, and strengthen the ability to perform personal life roles while increasing flexibility between roles.

The differences between psychodrama and drama therapy are not always clear. For me, they are analogous to the differences between ballet and modern dance. From the definition of drama therapy given above, one could say that psychodrama is a specialized form of drama therapy, even though drama therapy as a recognized therapeutic practice evolved after psychodrama. In truth, they both are current-day incarnations of ancient ritual and shamanistic practice.

One concrete difference between the two forms is the role of the director, or therapist. In psychodrama, the director almost never takes on a role within any scene. Even if psychodrama is being utilized with a single client, the director may voice a statement for a role, but generally does not enter into the action as a participant (*auxiliary*). In drama therapy, however, the director may often interact with a client or group members from within a role and/or as a co-creator of a dramatic improvisation.

Drama therapy may also make use of scripted theatre, assigning parts consciously to support therapeutic ends. In its infancy, much of drama therapy took this form. It is within the realm of sociodrama that Psychodrama and drama therapy become less distinguishable, although, once again, the role of the director may be the main indication.

I have been doing drama therapy since the days of the "Sex, Drugs, and Rock & Roll" project (see Introduction), although my formal training in the form did not begin until later. However, I consider myself a psychodramatist who also employs drama therapy methods, since the bulk of my training is in psychodrama. Interestingly, when asked by nontherapists what I do for work, I will generally say I am a drama therapist who works with teens. I have found that people who know nothing of either field can at least make a guess at what a drama therapist might be, while the term psychodramatist often evokes images of Alfred Hitchcock movies. As this book progresses, I will try to distinguish one form from another when the differences are significant.

Adolescence

A final term to be defined is adolescence, with respect to the ages included. I include preteens and young adults in the category of adolescence, and focus more on social context and maturity than on chronological age.

Why use action methods with adolescent groups?

I and other practitioners have found that action methods are ideally suited to many adolescent groups. Dramatic enactment or *role play* allows for "safe" experimentation with a wide range of social behaviors and situations as well as for practicing social skills. Working in a group setting with other adolescents provides both essential peer connections, as well as peer feedback. Since a major portion of the young person's life is spent in peer interaction, enactment within a peer group allows the process to mirror "real life" as well.

In recent decades, the focus on "science-based" programs with "measurable outcomes" has led to a great deal of research in youth prevention education, which has led, in turn, to the creation and marketing of a number of "prevention curricula." Although they may focus on different issues (e.g. HIV prevention or substance abuse prevention), their common goal is to decrease "high-risk behavior" in youth. These curricula have a number of things in common, among them: utilizing youth educators, particularly those who are a few years older than the group being educated; utilizing "action," rather than lecture/discussion alone; and using role play activities so that participants can "practice" positive skills and behaviors. Each of these factors has a parallel in the adolescent group.

The group experience can also help contain and direct the intensity of the adolescent experience. Just as Moreno described the toddler as operating within a state he called "megalomania normalis" (1959, p.139), a period of appropriate and normal egocentric perception, I propose that we view adolescence as a period of "histrionia normalis." Young people bring a great deal of intensity to their exploration of life and its complexities. Everything is amplified in intensity, and issues or happenings which to us, as adults, may seem insignificant carry great weight. Adolescence is naturally a time of extremes, and action techniques can provide an outlet for exploring these extremes in a safe and supported manner.

During this period of tremendous change, both physical and emotional, young people are also confronted with changing social demands and mixed messages. On the one hand, they are told "You're being childish!" On the other hand, the message is "You're not old enough, mature enough, or experienced enough!" Enactment can provide a safe outlet for expressing the frustrations of living with both internal and external conflicting demands.

Adolescents are also experimenting with finding their own identity while fitting into the group. Role play allows exploration of a wide range of behaviors and ways of being, as well as a rehearsal for the practical considerations of getting a job, or the interpersonal challenges of expressing feelings to a friend during a time of conflict.

Within the realm of practicing interpersonal skills, the action group provides a rich laboratory for experimenting with behaviors that will become vital in the selection of friends as well as life partners. Action approaches also help young people become more aware of the process of interaction and the changing nature of relationships as situations and personal circumstances change and develop. The entire range of social roles, from "popular kid" (*sociometric star*) to "loser" (*sociometric isolate*) can be explored (Moreno 1993).

Although he was writing about therapy in general, the following quote from Moreno and Moreno, about concepts which are discussed in greater detail later in this chapter, offers a compelling rationale for employing action approaches with adolescents:

> We live within the framework of time, space, and reality, but time learning, space learning, and reality learning cannot take place and be improved unless they are tested in an experimental setting, where they are experienced, expressed, practiced, and reintegrated within the framework of a psychotherapy which is modeled after life itself.... Thus it is imperative that we

transfer these phenomena from life itself into the therapeutic setting and back ... into life itself. (Moreno and Moreno 1975, p.22)

Adolescence provides a unique opportunity for revisiting the unmet developmental needs of childhood and reinforcing the foundation upon which adult roles will be built. Action methods are especially suited both for doing the repair work and for supporting the successful meeting of the challenges specific to adolescent development. Utilizing these approaches with adolescent groups, however, requires an understanding of the unique nature of the adolescent perspective. An appropriate framework within which to view this perspective is also found in the writings of J.L. Moreno and Zerka Moreno.

Moreno's universalia of psychotherapy

In *Psychodrama, Third Volume* (1975), Moreno and Moreno explored four principles that they called universalia of psychotherapy: *time, space, reality,* and *cosmos.* Although the term "universalia" implies an all-embracing truth, the manner in which various populations may relate to these truths will vary. In my experience, adolescents as a group encounter these universalia in a manner that is significantly different from most adults. Understanding the nature of these encounters is essential to doing any therapeutic work with adolescents, but this understanding is especially needed when utilizing action modalities.

Time

J.L. Moreno was interested in time as a therapeutic concept. Recognizing that an individual's health and pathology were inextricably connected to past, present, and future, he sought to "integrate all three dimensions into significant therapeutic operations" (Moreno and Moreno 1975, p.11). Moreno believed that Freud's emphasis on the past was too narrow. Moreno's view embraced bringing together "all three dimensions of time...in psychodrama, as they are in life, from the point of view of functional therapy" (p.13).

In working with adolescents, we indeed have to explore all three dimensions of time, and realize that young people seem to relate differently to each dimension from the ways most adults do. I begin my exploration of these differences with the adolescent perspective of "the past."

Adults may find it amusing and/or mysterious to hear teens talking about their childhoods as if they were "ancient history." To 15-year-olds, however, their 5-year-old lives are seen in that way. They lack perspective, or they may deliberately exaggerate this distance in their rush to claim their place as adults. This is especially true for those who have suffered from childhood abuse.

Victims of abuse may still be living in the same dysfunctional system within which the abuse took place, and so distancing themselves from the worst of it, or from the times in their lives when they felt most helpless within these traumatic settings, is a way of coping, one perhaps necessary to their survival. Viewing their younger childhood years as "a long time ago" is one way to accomplish this distancing. In this way, if the abuse, perhaps in a form more elusive than the legal definitions, may still be going on, the teens can view their younger, harsher years from a distance. Even yesterday or last week can be viewed as "quite a while ago" for this or other reasons, and may be a "do not touch" area for many teens.

Psychodrama has the potential for highly effective work in the area of recovery from trauma. However, it also has a tremendous potential to retraumatize. I explore the implications of this more fully in later chapters, but for the moment I will just post a sign that states: "Caution: Contents Extremely Hot." The past is not the place to start with adolescents. If the past is explored at all, it is only after working with young people to build sufficient skills and create adequate boundaries in the *present* so that they may return from a journey to the past more empowered than when they embarked.

As the past moves into the present, one notices that time appears to move differently for teens than it does for adults. Perhaps it is related to the fact that, for a 15-year-old, one year is a greater percentage of one's total life than it is to one who is 35.

As adults, we may smile at the young person who says, "I've been going out with him a long time. It's been three months now." Inwardly, we may be saying, "When you're as old as I am, you'll realize that three months is just a moment." The fact remains, however, that this young person is the client I am serving, so it is his/her perception of time that is relevant.

Adolescents operate within an "intensity of the moment" that most adults, for better or worse, have lost. I remember a young man I worked with some years ago who quipped, "I move around so fast, I think I'm going to be in the future before anyone else." Regardless of their speed, or at other times lethargy, it is in the present that adolescents allow themselves to be known. Unless we take the time to know them as they are, and meet them in that place with respect and without judgment, we cannot hope to support them in creating a more positive future.

As for the future, young people develop a more personal relationship to it as they approach young adulthood, and start to plan more consciously for moving toward it. Some may fantasize about a future in which things are better than at present, with no ideas for how to achieve such a future. For many, throughout much of their adolescence, however, the future is a vague "something" that belongs to adults who try to force them to prepare for it. For most, the functional future is tomorrow or next week.

We can support adolescents tremendously through training that focuses on the needs of the *immediate* future, but we must build skills in the present and not get too far ahead of ourselves. It is a good thing to equip young people with an expanded role repertoire for future use. However, models for many essential roles may not be found in their past experience. Our primary focus, therefore, must be on the present, as we help develop new roles and "new responses to old situations," which is part of Moreno's definition of "spontaneity" (1964, p.50).

From within the "Here and Now and all its immediate personal, social and cultural implications" (Moreno and Moreno 1975, p.12), we can support young people in creating a *functional present*. This can, in turn, aid them in moving beyond the dysfunctions of the past, as well as in opening new possibilities for the future.

Space

In exploring the concept of space, Moreno reflected that, in a psychoanalytic office, the space is not related to the therapeutic process, while "psychodrama, which is action centered...tries to integrate all the dimensions of living into itself" (Moreno and Moreno 1975, pp.13–14). The use of scene setting and the exploration of material in action encourage kinesthetic involvement in the therapeutic process. Although these are of value to any group member, regardless of age, the integration of movement with cognition is especially important for adolescents. This form of therapeutic group work provides a venue within which those who have difficulty articulating what they are thinking or feeling, and those who have difficulty sitting still, can still participate fully.

Although Moreno talked about space primarily in terms of creating psychodramatic scenes and placing them in an actual context (the living room of the house, with walls of a certain color, and windows situated on certain walls, etc.), in working with adolescents, *inner space* becomes just as important as external reality. Much of the psychodramatic work that teens create is *intrapsychic* in nature, generated while opposing thoughts or feelings dialogue with each other, or different aspects of self get together to renegotiate their relationship to the protagonist. This internal landscape is as important and real a setting as any living room. The manner in which young people relate to external reality is, of course, also significant.

Young people can, paradoxically, both claim space and give it up in the same instant. They will argue over whose chair it is, push and shove to claim the choice spot, and then end up draping body parts over each other as they sit in proximity. Their childhood sense of territoriality ("That's mine!") is maturing into a more communal view, but the process is not always a smooth one.

If we are committed to creating space that is related to the therapeutic process, then we do well to invite our adolescent group members to become, as much as possible, co-creators of the space in which they will work. I have heard theories extolling the virtue of relatively bland and sterile environments as less distracting for therapeutic work. I do prefer a space with no windows through which outsiders may peek, but the benefits of a space in which young people feel ownership and thereby safe, comfortable and at home, far outweigh what little benefit may be provided by a so-called sterile, or neutral environment. For many, there is no safe space in their outside world, and the one we create, within which our group's work will be conducted, is an invaluable aspect of the therapeutic process.

Reality

Moreno described three types of reality: *reduced*, or *infra-reality*; *life*, or *actual reality*; and *surplus reality* (Moreno and Moreno 1975, p.15). It is important, once again, to view each in relation to its potential meanings to an adolescent.

INFRA-REALITY

Infra-reality refers to the reality in a therapist's office, within which the contact is "not a genuine dialog, but sort of an interview, a research situation or projection test" (Moreno and Moreno 1975, p.15). In order to function well in this type of setting, one generally needs to be more comfortable with higher levels of cognition, to be engaging more frequently in abstract thinking, and to be more capable and willing to sit in one place for 50 minutes than many adolescents are. Research in recent years on the physiological development of the brain during adolescence, as well as recognition of the developmental task of moving from concrete to abstract thinking and its usual occurrence during, rather than before, adolescence, lead to the conclusion that infra-reality is not "where it's at" for most teens.

ACTUAL REALITY

Actual reality, of course, refers to the way people live their day-to-day lives. Moreno and Moreno (1975) pointed out that this reality may not always be satisfactory or desired. However, even though the individual may want to change, rigid patterns evolved over time, along with fear of moving into an unknown situation, may prohibit change. For the adolescent, actual reality is, in many ways, more rigid than for adults. The power to make decisions, change laws, proscribe and punish behaviors all lies in the hands of adults. Moving from the perception that "life is something that happens to me" to "life is something I participate in creating" is a major developmental task, and one at which many do not succeed, even after adolescence.

As therapists and youth workers, we must be cognizant of the actual realities of the uses of parental consent, the enforcement of current laws about reporting actual or suspected cases of abuse, and the ways our juvenile justice systems often focus on changing behaviors rather than on supporting healthy development. We must also be aware that many of the young people with whom we work may live in situations that are quite devastating, though not "legally" abusive or negligent, and that these young people are not at liberty to move or find a better situation. An adolescent's ability as well as opportunity to manipulate his or her actual reality is still developing and requires our support. One of the ways we can support their ability to cope with actual reality is to offer opportunities to try out other ways of living and responding in surplus reality.

SURPLUS REALITY

Surplus reality, simply stated, is the reality we create because the actual reality in which we find ourselves is not adequate or sufficient for our needs. Moreno (1944) described it thus:

> When God created the world in six days he had stopped a day too early. He had given Man a place to live but in order to make it safe for him he also chained him to that place. On the seventh day he should have created for Man a second world, another one, free of the first world and in which he could purge himself from it, but a world which would not chain anyone because it was not real. It is here where the theatre of spontaneity continues God's creation of the world by opening for Man a new dimension of existence. (p.7)

It is within the realm of surplus reality that psychodrama occurs. Moreno used the term to refer to a wide range of psychodramatic techniques, including *role reversal*, *role training*, and *role playing*, as auxiliaries in another's drama. He stated: "There are certain invisible dimensions in the reality of living, not fully experienced or expressed, and that is why we have to use surplus operations and surplus instruments to bring them out in our therapeutic settings" (Moreno and Moreno 1975, p.16). Each of the above-named techniques is uniquely suited to assisting teens with the developmental tasks of adolescence.

Role reversal

In role reversal, the protagonist does not merely stand in another's role, or pretend to be another, but is enjoined "to try and feel his way into the thinking, feeling, and behavior patterns of the other" (Moreno and Moreno 1975, p.16). First, the role is played by the protagonist according to his or her perceptions. Then an auxiliary takes the role, as presented, and allows the protagonist to switch back and forth between the roles and perspectives of "self" and "other." This is an essential step in developing a more mature sense of empathy. Since the role reversals occur in surplus reality rather than actual reality, the protagonist and auxiliaries are safe to explore feelings and insights throughout these experiences.

Role training

In role training, the protagonist can try on new or emerging roles, explore different ways of playing current roles, or work on eliminating the maladaptive behaviors that manifest regularly in particular roles. A key element of role training is that, again because of the deployment of surplus reality, the protagonist is free to make mistakes and learn from them without having to suffer the consequences of actual reality mistakes. This provides an ideal setting for integrating consequential thinking, one of the tasks in the development of the functioning of the adolescent brain.

Role playing

In role playing, as an auxiliary in another's drama, one puts aside one's own needs, thoughts, and perceptions and exists in service to another. Each of these experiences serves the young person in moving from the self-centered world of the child, through the other-centered world of the adolescent, and into the self-in-relation-to-others world of the healthy, mature adult.

In addition to describing the setting of psychodramatic technique, surplus reality also describes the world of imagination, of fantasy, of delusion. From this perspective, adolescents dwell in surplus reality most of the time. I do not mean this statement as derogatory, but as a celebration of the intensity of the reality through which young people experience life. Events have greater value and emotions have more intensity for most adolescents than they seem to for most adults. It may be a result, as current neurobiological research suggests, of a swelling and increasingly active amygdala within the limbic area of the brain coupled with hormonal surges, but this intensity provides both motivation and energy for learning about life. It is a part of the developing ability to discern and discriminate, to be able to recognize that the loss of a family heirloom is a greater loss than that of a favorite CD.

Adolescents' perspectives of the world, though colored greatly by their experiences, needs, and feelings of the moment, become their views of actual reality, whether or not these are views that anyone else shares. Learning and understanding that others have different and also valid perspectives on the same event are significant milestones. Even events that we, as adults, may consider bald-faced lies ("I didn't hit him!") may, sometimes, more accurately be manifestations of an ability to create an alternative reality on the spot and firmly believe in it. Although frustrating to those of us who work with young people, it is a normal and healthy part of the adolescent transition to reshape reality in this manner.

Cosmos

Moreno's view of the cosmos is central to his philosophy and has been reflected upon by a number of Morenian scholars. In his chapter in the book, *Psychodrama since Moreno* (1994), Jonathan Moreno reflected on his father's response to the cosmic, existential dilemma. I would summarize Jonathan's reflection thus: If the only choices we have are to subscribe to the ultimate meaninglessness of everything or to become God, then let's become God. When one embraces universality, then responsibility follows.

In 1909, at age 20, J.L. Moreno penned *The Words of the Father* (1941), as legend has it, in a moment of spontaneous inspiration, using red ink, and writing on the attic walls. This was his first articulation of his developing understanding of the relationship between humanity and the Godhead. He was not speaking of the "*He* God" of the Hebrews, omniscient and omnipotent; nor of the "*Thou* God" of the Christians, all-loving and forgiving. Moreno, choosing existential jubilation over existential despair, claimed his participation in the "I God," expressed in the world through spontaneity and creativity.

If we embrace this philosophy, it may lead us to muse something like this: If I am co-creator, an integral piece of God and all creation, then I must have at my disposal the means to create, to relate, and to accept responsibility for self and others. This philosophy, whether taken literally or metaphorically, can help create a firm foundation for the adolescent's journey from an external to an internal sense of control and responsibility.

Moreno's reclaiming of the cosmic relationship as an integral part of his philosophy, during a time in which "science" was trying to push "religion" to the side, makes psychodrama a powerful tool for working with adolescents. Many young people, as they move from childhood's acceptance of what they have been told and taught and begin to question the often confusing religious beliefs of their parents or community, are looking for a genuine sense of the *transpersonal*, something beyond the self, in which they can believe. Others, for whom childhood was a time of no religious or spiritual training, experience the lack of the transpersonal as contributing to an unidentified longing. Some, who have been victims of ritual abuse, cannot fathom anything of value or safety outside the self.

There is a tremendous drive during adolescence to find meaning and purpose in life. The manner in which the needs to reconnect to and explore the cosmic are met has a significant impact on the ways adolescents will conduct their personal, family, social, and community lives as they move into adulthood.

Moreno and Moreno (1975) defined the cosmic in terms not only of the religious and spiritual, but also in terms of other universals of living, including age, gender, destiny, belief, and heritage. All of these elements play a part in the adolescent's discovery of personal identity, and all can be explored from any perspective on the psychodrama stage. Males and females can take on each other's roles; the young can play the old and vice versa. We can talk to God, and God can respond.

The degree to which open discussion of the cosmic may be appropriate to a particular group of adolescents, and the degree to which issues of faith and spirituality become part of the transpersonal perspective, may well vary in different cultures, and even within specific communities in a given culture. It remains vital, however, for young people to have a supported venue for cosmic exploration.

Summary

As therapists and counselors, we have a unique opportunity to provide a healing experience when we work with adolescent groups. Action techniques allow us to work effectively and efficiently with young people, to respect them for who they are, and to offer support for their journey. It is vital to have a strong philosophical frame, as well as a theoretical one, in order to bring integrity and purpose to our work with adolescents. My understanding of Moreno's philosophy, articulated in this chapter, has provided a richly appropriate frame in my work.

As we embrace our service to young people, and allow ourselves to see the world through their eyes, we help them become empowered to choose and to learn from their choices. It is the ability to choose that is vital. Choices will sometimes be mistaken, but that too is part of the learning process.

In Chapter 2, I offer a theoretical foundation for understanding adolescent group development as well as the developmental challenges of the adolescent members that can be addressed in a group setting.

Viewing Adolescence from a Developmental Perspective

In this chapter I explore development, beginning with the parallel process of group development as it relates to individual development in infancy and early childhood. Understanding these parallels helps us to understand more fully the needs of the group and its members as they progress from the *beginning stage* through the *transition stage* into the *working stage* and on to *termination*. There are a number of valid frameworks from which to view group development. I have chosen this simple one because my goal is to focus on adolescents and action techniques, and not create another book on understanding group development.

Once this foundation has been laid, I will explore the specific developmental tasks of adolescence and the ways in which group process can support their accomplishment. I also present an overview of the continuum of developmental change that occurs across sequential age clusters within the adolescent years.

I considered having as a title for this chapter: "The Quest for Object Constancy through Group Dynamics, or, Getting Past the Transition Stage," but it seemed a bit cumbersome, although appropriately descriptive. My theoretical framework borrows concepts from ego psychology as expressed in the writing of Eric Erikson (1950), and object relations theory as expressed by Mahler *et al.* (1975), with just a touch of D.W. Winnicott (1958) and Jean B. Miller (1986) thrown in for good measure. Although, with the exception of Miller, these theorists may be a bit "old school," I employ their concepts to help create a useful construct with which to view the material. Miller's (1986) work is probably most relevant to the way I have come to utilize these concepts in adolescent groups. I begin with a few basic assumptions:

1. The stages through which a group develops parallel the developmental stages of the individual in infancy and early childhood.

2.   Developmental stages are cumulative, in that unless the tasks of the
      earlier stages are successfully completed, the challenges of the later
      stages cannot be fully met.

3.   Although cumulative, the stages are not strictly linear, that is, there is
      a great deal of overlap and moving back and forth between the
      developmental tasks as the individuals or group move forward.

4.   In successfully negotiating the developmental stages of the group, we
      can provide a "corrective emotional experience" for members who did
      not fully master the developmental challenges in their individual lives.

5.   In order for a group to move into the working stage, it must achieve
      the group equivalent of object constancy.

Stages and phases of group development

Given these assumptions and the existing parallels that are evident between group
process and individual development, we can explore further the changing needs,
challenges, and tasks of each stage of group development, for members as well as
leaders.

The beginning stage

The beginning or *forming* stage of a group actually begins before the group has
started. Members generally go through some kind of information, application and
selection process. It is here that members first deal with the critical issues of the
beginning stage, which are trust and safety, and which continue once the group
has formed and is running. Members must deal with their fears of not being
accepted by others in the group. They must get to know each other and themselves
in relation to the group and other members. I can remember initial group sessions
in which potential members considered whether or not they could remain in the
group because of prior history with other members.

Erikson (1950) calls his first stage of individual development *Trust vs. Mistrust*,
which certainly parallels the prime focus of the group's beginning stage. Mahler *et
al.* (1975) subdivides this first developmental stage into three segments. The first
she calls the *Symbiotic*, in which the child and mother are closely merged. This is
paralleled by the leader-dependent nature of the first part of the beginning stage.
By attaching themselves to the group, other members, and the group leader(s),
members ward off anxiety. The tasks are primarily interpersonal in nature as
members check for safety, consistency, and containment. The development of

clear group norms to which members can agree to adhere is essential to this stage of development.

Mahler *et al.*'s (1975) second stage is called *Differentiation*. At this point, the child's awareness of the "me" and the "not me" becomes more fully developed. Body boundaries become more clearly delineated, and although still dependent, the child recognizes self as separate from the caregiver. This seems to parallel the second phase of the beginning stage of group as well. Members are starting to feel more comfortable with the group, each other, and the leader(s), and individual issues start to come to the fore. With the *inter*personal safely established, the *intra*personal can begin to emerge.

The "everything is wonderful" ambiance that generally permeates initial group sessions may start to fade. Anxiety becomes more evident and resistance may appear, evidenced by members not paying attention or fooling around. Conflict may begin to emerge between members, and some may even leave the group, although a general sense of order still prevails.

I should clarify, at this point, that my experience has been primarily with voluntary groups, with members participating because they wanted to be there, or quickly deciding that it was not the place for them and leaving. With compulsory groups, the process is often different, and getting members to the point of recognizing that the group is a good and safe place can take considerable effort, and more time.

I should also reiterate the third assumption. Clearly stages and phases are artificial categories that we cannot take too literally. They overlap and interweave, and different members move at different speeds and in different ways. The sequence of development, however general, does hold as a basic framework from which to observe the group's process, although the pattern often fluctuates and sometimes the group moves back a few degrees before surging forward.

Mahler *et al.*'s (1975) next subphase is called *Practicing*, and is the beginning of what she describes as the separation/individuation process. It is marked by the infant's moving away from the caregiver for gradually increasing periods with frequent returns for "emotional refueling." In a group, this is evidenced by an increasing sense of individual identity in the members and by more overt testing of the structure and the leaders. It is, in a way, a rehearsal for the transition stage.

The transition stage

This stage of group development is marked by an increase in anxiety and defensiveness by members (and sometimes by leaders as well). Fears of looking foolish, of being rejected if one really opens oneself, of losing control, etc., come more strongly into play, often on an unconscious level. Resistance may increase, as may control issues. Conflicts between members and struggle with the authority of the leader(s) may emerge. Yalom (1995) points out that these issues are often a recapitulation of the primary family experience; within a safe therapeutic group, members have the opportunity to "correct" the experience.

Langs (1981) refers to this phenomenon as *Secure Frame Dread*. The therapeutic container has been carefully constructed, so members begin to feel the imminence of significant disclosure within an environment in which it is actually safe to disclose significant personal material. The old "reptilian brain" kicks in and the message (generally subconscious) is received: "Flee!"

The parallels at this point to individual development are most illuminating. Erikson (1950) calls this stage of development *Autonomy vs. Shame and Doubt*, with the child's major tasks being the development of self-control (both physical and emotional) and will power. Mahler *et al.* (1975) calls this subphase of the separation/individuation process *Rapprochement*. The child's focus becomes a developing sense of autonomy, along with the ability to say "No!"

The overlapping nature of the stages and the manner in which they melt into each other are, as noted, sometimes misleading. *Rapprochement/Transition* does not appear full-blown and in a particular instant. Just as the infant develops incrementally, so, too, within the transition stage of the group, uncertainty moves gradually into anxiety, concerns into fears, and questions into challenges.

My understanding of development has been greatly influenced by the basic principles of relational therapy, as espoused by Jean Baker Miller (1986) and others. Traditional models of human development generally focus on the male child, and, in reality, our social expectations of children's appropriate development is gender biased. Boys are enculturated to follow the path of separation/individuation while girls are given the task of maintaining relationship. The ensuing potential for conflict has been the subject of many popular books.

A less gender-biased perspective views the challenges at each stage of development in terms of moving toward "more mature relationship" (Miller 1986). I find this view especially enlightening as a group leader in working creatively and nonjudgmentally with behaviors that occur during the transition stage of group development.

It is unreasonable to single out one stage as more important than all the others, especially since they are interdependent and usually overlapping, but, in the life of the individual as well as of the group, this is certainly a crucial time. Many individuals and groups never successfully negotiate these stormy seas. One reason may be that this is the most difficult stage for the caregiver/group leader. Tending the child/group with love and care at each stage is a challenge. It is easier, however, when the child/group is sweet, dependent, responsive and (essentially) easily controlled. Deep fears, uncertainties, and insecurities can be triggered for us as adults when the adorable and adoring child or group begins to resist, to separate, to claim his/her/their individuality, to say "No!"

This is the point at which the parallel between Winnicott's (1958) "good-enough" parent and the "good-enough" group leader becomes especially informative. The good-enough parent allows autonomous action while still providing guidance, support, and protection. The good-enough group leader attends with honesty to the emerging "shadows" and allows and supports the conflict and challenges to move into the light, rather than ignoring, resisting, or trying to control them with increased authoritarian fervor based on fears of losing control of the group. Despite the mandates of managed care, the courts, or the parents, therapists and group leaders who work with young people serve best by letting go of the desire to manage behavior, and focusing on fostering the building of more mature relationships, which allows group members and their group to move appropriately into the next stage.

The working stage

The working stage is to the group's development what *object constancy* is to the individual's development. Object constancy, in object relations theory, is the result of the successful negotiation through the earlier stages of development (Mahler *et al.* 1975). The child has developed a sense of safety and trust, has learned to distinguish the "me" from the "not me," has had the opportunity to experiment with independent action while under the protective supervision of the caregiver, and has developed a sense of self which is capable of valuable independent action apart from the caregiver. She or he has internalized the *object*, and then is ready to move on to new areas of growth, exploration, and learning (Mahler *et al.* 1975).

So, too, can the group develop an internalized sense of safety and trust (*group cohesion*) which allows members to appreciate the universality of their life issues, and to give and receive support to and from one another in working through their issues. Members are increasingly able to be vulnerable with each other, to comfort others with care and concern, to state more clearly and specifically their individual and group goals, and to risk disclosing personal material. There is a sense of belonging and a sense of hope.

Erikson (1950) calls the parallel individual developmental stage *Initiative vs. Guilt*, and notes that this stage includes both direction and purpose. The child is developing self-control, is learning to plan successfully, and is feeling sufficiently empowered to undertake the challenge of conquering the environment. As a group successfully negotiates the working stage, the members have had the opportunity to correct some of the negative experiences that may have prevented them from successfully completing this stage in their individual development. The group can now encounter the challenge of negotiating appropriate and healthy closure as the sessions come to an end.

Termination

All groups must end, or at the very least, within the life of the group, membership changes. Termination as a group's stage includes all issues related to endings, long-lasting change of membership, and any leaders leaving. For the group, issues of termination and ending (hopefully) come significantly sooner than for the individual. Even in long-term groups, issues of *termination anxiety* may arise early in the process and become more evident as the group reaches the end of its time together. (The comparison to infant and child development is less direct at this point, but is perhaps seen in the *separation anxiety* many children experience, which often occurs when a parent leaves, or the child goes to childcare or school.) Termination issues are a true test of object constancy: will the sense of safety, belonging, and ability to work though adversity last after the group is no longer meeting, or after the composition of the group membership changes?

The same processes that Elisabeth Kübler-Ross (1971) discusses in her work on death and dying come into play as a group is ending: *anger, denial, bargaining, grief,* and *acceptance.* Once again, the leader supports group members in expressing and examining their feelings and moving through these phases.

Members may feel anger at the leaders: "If you really cared about us, you wouldn't end the group." Denial may be evident in a number of ways: "We'll see each other around, so it's not really over," or "This group wasn't so special anyhow." Members may try to bargain or negotiate for extending the group.

With support and sufficient time given to the process, the members will be able to express their grief and sadness to each other as well as to offer important feedback and appreciations to each other and the leader(s). The group can then end with acceptance and the knowledge that, while this group may be over, there will be other life experiences with the potential for being equally rewarding and challenging.

Certainly, when I left ACTINGOUT (see the Introduction for the background on this program), we spent a good part of my final year dealing with termination with the older members with whom I had relationships lasting many years. For many of them, I had become the "good father" who had never been in their lives before. This was an issue we had always addressed openly in the group, with my having "officially" accepted the role for some members, along with a clear contract of what this role meant. My impending departure stimulated feelings of desertion and abandonment that manifested in some members as anger, in others as denial, and in others as regression. It was imperative that the group become even more aware of the process so that together we could identify the roles I held for each of them and they could each claim these roles back into their own role repertoires. Details of this process are given in Chapter 8.

The issues faced by the group during the transition stage and during termination are, in many ways, also related to the developmental tasks of adolescence itself, with its own array of challenges to be met, obstacles to be overcome, and victories to be claimed.

The developmental tasks of adolescence

A positive group experience can provide immeasurable support to adolescents in negotiating the developmental challenges of the teen years. For the purpose of this exploration, I first provide an overview of these challenges, and then, later in the chapter, review some of the more specific substages along the developmental continuum during the adolescent years. In this overview, I divide the developmental tasks and challenges into general categories of *personal, interpersonal,* and *transpersonal,* and explore the range of issues that are encountered over time in each of these areas.

The personal

During adolescence, the child generally experiences rapid changes in physical size, shape, and functioning. The endocrine system begins working overtime and hormones surge through the body. New pathways are being developed in the brain at an amazing rate, allowing new kinds of thought processes to take place. By the time young people reach the age of 20, they have generally grown into their adult bodies. In the best of environments and with the healthiest of children, the mere physical changes associated with adolescence provide challenges of their own. A supportive group experience helps normalize the growing experience and provides a forum for discussion and information gathering.

The world of emotions becomes more complex, as the young person experiences blended feelings and fine shades of difference within feelings previously experienced as more black or white. The group provides a venue within which to learn to express affect. In addition, as the ability to become self-critical develops, the group provides a reality check, offering the opportunity to see self through another's eyes. The young person begins to develop the ability to observe from outside of the affect, and without judgment.

Piaget (1963) named the adolescent stage of intellectual development *Formal Operations*. With concomitant neural development, the ability for abstract thought emerges, along with the ability to understand the personal perception of reality as one of many possible views. The ability to see consequences is also developing: "If I do such-and-such, then a possible outcome is…" Although these changes are happening within the individual, it is through social interchange that young people discover and integrate these personal changes.

The interpersonal

There are some who argue that, at this point in development, the peer group becomes more important than the family or community. I would argue that it is more useful to think in terms of differences in role function. The roles of the peer group in providing support and a sense of commonality of experience are crucial to survival. However, as the role of the family shifts, the presence of other positive adults who can help provide a cognitive structure within which communicative exchange can happen enhances the young person's ability to discover his or her adult self. Research has demonstrated the importance of positive, caring adults in developing resilient youth (Resnick *et al.* 1997). Adults not only provide caring relationships with young people, but also provide a template for cognitive development that is not provided by peers, as vital as peer relationships are. Adults support young people in learning how to discover and articulate the meaning that comes from experience.

Adolescence is also a rehearsal period for adult relationships, whether as friends, employees, colleagues, or lovers, with lessons in trust and betrayal, challenges to authority, and the transitory nature of many relationships. As group members deal with the struggles of moving through the transition stage and working through the feelings that come with termination issues, they are developing skills and roles that will enable them to be more healthy adults, capable of more mature relationships.

The transpersonal

A major part of the task of "making meaning" for adolescents falls within the realm of the transpersonal, as young people struggle to comprehend that which is greater than self. Whether it is approached from the philosophical or the spiritual, the cultural or the social, the sublime or the ridiculous, young people seek to discover the "meaning of life." Moreno referred to this dimension of exploration as cosmos (see Chapter 1). Once again, the support of peers, with recognition of common experience, and the cognitive frame provided by the adult leader provide a safe container within which the exploration can proceed.

Children generally accept the cultural, religious, and spiritual beliefs of their parents without question and, often, without understanding. It is during adolescence that young people begin to question and challenge what they have been taught. Although religious education is not an appropriate goal of a therapy group, the spiritual dimension of group members' lives should not be avoided.

I will explore personal, interpersonal, and transpersonal adolescent developmental challenges and the skills needed to meet them more thoroughly using the Therapeutic Spiral Model™ (Hudgins 2002) as a frame of reference in Chapter 3. Additionally, I will be introducing the concepts of *observation* and *containment* as further categories of adolescent developmental challenges. In Chapter 7, I provide a range of activities to support these personal, interpersonal, transpersonal, observational, and containment developmental tasks.

At this point, however, it is important to recognize that the adolescent years contain a range of experiences and developmental challenges. Therefore, I offer this more detailed view of the continuum of adolescent development.

The developmental continuum of adolescence

Just as adolescents present significantly different challenges to the group leader than adults do, so do the challenges vary along the adolescent age continuum. For the purposes of this exploration, I will consider "early" adolescence to be somewhere around 11 to 13 years of age; "mid"-adolescence 14 to 16 years; "late" adolescence 17 to 19 years; and "young adult" 20 to 25 years. Consider the words and numbers to be convenient descriptors of common behavior clusters even though different young people develop at different rates.

To provide some sort of frame and continuity, I further divide this exploration into the areas of *physical, mental, emotional, personal,* and *social development.* Again, the linear limits of language may separate the discussion of these categories, while, in reality, their effects are interactive.

Physical development

The changes in physical development from early to late adolescence are dramatic, as puberty begins and myriad internal and external changes occur. There is also a resurgence of brain development during adolescence. The midbrain, the center for relationship and emotional significance, undergoes a sudden growth spurt brought on by hormonal changes. The frontal cortex is also sending out new neurons and discarding those that do not prove significant as it develops its capacity for higher level functioning.

EARLY ADOLESCENCE

The physical changes of puberty during early adolescence, though perhaps eagerly awaited, can also undermine or threaten the sense of self that has remained relatively stable for a while. Puberty is a time during which many young people are teased about how quickly or slowly they are developing. Girls who are first among their peers to menstruate and/or develop breasts can be both envied and scorned. The same can be true for boys in terms of genital growth, voice changes, and facial hair.

MID-ADOLESCENCE

Young people at this age are still growing and changing a great deal. They usually become more concerned with body and appearance, judging themselves against perceived norms presented by peers and in the media. Issues with facial complexion have begun for many. Problems with weight and/or height are significant in many cultures. Most females and some males are fully grown during this stage.

LATE ADOLESCENCE

By this point in time, most males and all females are in the final stages of growing into their adult bodies. They look adult and, for some aspects in the USA, become "legally" adult at age 18 (can vote, be drafted, enter into contracts, be considered a legal adult for all courts). Neural growth within the brain is generally winding down, but not quite complete. Physical appearance becomes even more important as pressures to be partnered increase.

YOUNG ADULT

By this point, the physical growth, including neural development, is completed. Young people must come to terms with long-term appearance issues, such as height, body type, and facial complexion. They become "fully adult" in all legal ways in the USA at age 21.

In dealing with issues of physical development, it may be helpful for group leaders to have books available about the growth process or access to information that members may not be getting from other sources. All of the physical issues mentioned above may be brought as concerns to the group. As members' ages increase, fears about "how I will turn out" transform into issues of self-acceptance.

For groups in which members are relatively homogeneous in age, the leader may be an important source of support. In groups with mixed age membership, the older members may offer support to the younger ones, although they may require support in doing this in a constructive rather than teasing manner.

Adolescent development, of course, is not just a physical matter. Mental capacity is also developing along with bodies and brains.

Mental development

Mental development is significant during adolescence, both as a result of neural development in the frontal cortex as well as societal expectations and pressures, especially for academic success. Certain capacities are developing, such as those for abstract thought and for being able to deal with multiple tasks at the same time. Parents and teachers may have unrealistic expectations about the young person's readiness for specific tasks and responsibilities. Enhanced midbrain activity (see Emotional development, p.46) may interfere with cortical functioning.

EARLY ADOLESCENCE

This period marks the bridge between concrete and abstract thought, as young people become increasingly articulate, logical, critical, and interested. It takes time to move from "black and white" thinking to appreciation of the "shades of gray." The simultaneous tremendous activity within both the midbrain and frontal cortex can often lead to confusion. Imagination is transforming from that of the child to that of the adult, and may seem a bit stifled at this point.

MID-ADOLESCENCE

By this point, young people are (generally) fully in abstract thought, and can plan for and imagine a future for themselves, as tentative as this process may be. Abilities to multitask are increasing. Because of the young people's physical maturity, adults may expect adult behavior; yet the finer mental capacities are still developing, so this development requires support as well as adult modeling. Imagination is more fully linked to creativity by this point and creative inspiration is rampant.

LATE ADOLESCENCE

Young people will generally think of themselves as fully "grown up" by this point, but, in fact, the fine tuning in cortical development is still going on. At this age, however, the mental skills are well enough developed that creative output can be quite startling, and the artists, poets, musicians, dancers, and inventors have generally begun to emerge.

YOUNG ADULT

With cortical functions fully in place, all capacities are available. Provided they have had some significant supportive experiences during the earlier years, reason and logic as well as creativity are fully functioning. The only thing lacking is length of experience.

During this time of significant mental development, adults can provide important models of higher level cortical functioning, including the ability to make meaning from experience. It is important for group leaders to understand, appreciate, and work with the subtleties of mental development in order to provide reasonable expectations as well as appropriate boundaries and containment.

Disparities in mental development make it difficult to run groups that contain members who are both in early and late adolescence. Older members often become impatient with the younger. My recommendation is for more homogeneous groupings in terms of age. When a wide mix of ages is present, tactics such as pairing younger and older members for special mentoring activities or offering subgroupings within which members can engage in certain experiences with those they consider "peers" can both prove helpful.

As the body and mind develop, so do the presence of and capacity to be affected by the emotions.

Emotional development

Unlike physical growth, which requires only nourishment, appropriate physical stimulation, and the unfolding of a genetic code, emotional growth is dependent on experience as well. The interactions with peer groups play a large part, but so do family interactions as well as the social structures and strictures within which the young person develops. There is significant activity in the midbrain during adolescence. The amygdala, prompted by hormonal changes, swells and becomes more active. It is the center for assigning emotional significance to experience, and is responsible for much of the emotional intensity of adolescence. Understanding that this intensity, including a propensity for aggressive behavior, is neuro-physiologically based is important in creating a nonjudgmental therapeutic environment.

Although sexual development could easily be included in any of the categories I am using in this exploration, I will include it here, since it certainly is related to emotional intensity as well as to feelings that can often preoccupy a young person.

EARLY ADOLESCENCE

During this time, young people crave, yet reject and/or feel embarrassed by emotion and physical closeness, attention, and touch. Many intense and oppositional, quickly changing feelings (some sexual) are felt. Questions regarding sexual and/or gender identity arise during this age, and even earlier, but often are not discussed. Societal pressures to be romantically involved may not correspond to actual feelings, but young people may be more inclined to follow the crowd than the urgings of their own bodies. Combine this with the mental confusion discussed earlier, and this period certainly can make a claim for the title of "most difficult part of adolescence."

Many older adolescents, reflecting back on this period, will recall it as the most difficult. Then, they will be quick to add that the rest doesn't necessarily become easier, just a little less hard.

MID-ADOLESCENCE

By this point, most young people are becoming more introspective and less quick to react, with fewer oppositional emotions. Feelings are still intense, although perhaps not quite so confusing or unfathomable. Sexual feelings are very prevalent and may be acted upon. Again, social pressures for partnering may prompt some to engage in sexual activity before they feel they are ready. Issues of sexual and gender identity and activity are prominent and become considered more seriously.

Adolescents at this age are often torn between wanting to fit in and be accepted by peers and wanting to develop their own identities. Being in a space of "in between," no longer a child and not quite an adult, can exacerbate intense feelings of isolation.

LATE ADOLESCENCE

Emotionally, adolescents at this age are generally very independent, although usually still financially dependent upon others. This can certainly contribute to feelings of frustration as well as anxiety as they begin to contemplate becoming self-supporting. The need to fit in has generally diminished somewhat by this point, but ambivalent feelings about letting go of childhood may become more conscious. If individuals have received appropriate support in younger years, their ability to contain emotions has increased.

Young people are probably sexually active by this age. Those who are gay, lesbian, bisexual, transgendered, or transsexual are having a harder time maintaining self-denial, if that had been a way of dealing with earlier feelings. Those who were earlier aware of their sexual orientation or gender minority status, but did not get support or feel safe enough to seek it earlier, will often look for opportunities to find support during these years.

YOUNG ADULT

As young people move out on their own, off to higher education or whatever situation in which they intend to live, issues of self-worth and competence come to the fore. They may feel hopeful or hopeless about the future; these feelings may be based on life situations more than on fear or imagination. Sexuality is, hopefully, an integrated aspect of self and life.

If they have been well supported during their adolescence, young people generally find a degree of emotional maturity at this point. If not, then emotional difficulties have the potential for resulting in significant problems, including absenteeism from work, substance abuse and addiction, anti-social behavior, domestic violence, and subsequent incarceration. Those with mental disorders are generally experiencing them in full, by this point, and, if fortunate, have been diagnosed and are receiving treatment.

Within the realm of emotional development, the group experience can have tremendous significance. Knowing they are not alone in their feelings is important for young people at any age. The group can also provide a safe place within which to fully experience what one is feeling and explore different ways of expressing feelings. Action techniques, such as role playing, allow experimentation with ways of expressing feelings and trying on "unhealthy" behaviors without having to face the consequences.

Similar concerns about age groupings come from the discrepancy between levels of emotional maturity as young people progress along the continuum. Homogeneous age groupings are likely to be more satisfactory for participants. Leaders who conduct groups for several different age clusters need to spend part of their warm-up to each group session reflecting on and connecting to the emotional tone of the members of that particular group.

As young people develop physically, mentally, and emotionally, the adult personality begins to emerge.

Personal development

It is difficult to separate "personal" development from the other elements being discussed, but for the purposes of this exploration, the phrase will relate primarily to the development of a sense of personal identity and personality. As will be discussed in Chapter 7, Moreno contended that the self emerges from the roles we play (Moreno 1964), and so, from this perspective, the development of the adolescent self as well as the adolescent's developing perception of self are related to the increases in role experience and role demands during this period. Both internal and external forces make demands on the adolescent to change and increase the role repertoire during the transition from child to adult.

EARLY ADOLESCENCE

As they begin adolescence, young people are trying to balance the need for independence with the need for adult advocacy and involvement. Childhood roles like the "carefree player" and the "watched over youngster" begin to be exchanged for roles like the "engaged student" and the "independent explorer." The young person begins to define self in a more autonomous manner from family and in a more connected manner with peers.

MID-ADOLESCENCE

As they get a little older, young people begin looking for a sense of self as being needed and important to others and to causes. They seek more responsibility and independence. The roles of "trusted friend" and "independent thinker" become more important, while roles of the "obedient child" or "loving son or daughter" generally become less significant.

LATE ADOLESCENCE

As they approach young adulthood, young people generally have an established moral code, although they may not always follow it. Issues about the present and the future begin to combine and young people begin to have a personal sense of history. The role of the "rebel with a cause" is well established at this point, as are the "leaver behind of childhood" and the "stepper into the future." Roles of "trusted employee" or "hopelessly unemployable" are also emerging.

YOUNG ADULT

As they reach this point, young people are generally evaluating which roles they will take with them into their adult lives and which they must leave behind in childhood or adolescence. Social roles relating to job and career and partnered relationship move into the forefront.

Groups and their leaders can also provide tremendous support during this time of personal development. The leader needs to consider the differing needs within the age clusters. For example, the early adolescents need fairness, consistency, firmness, structure, clarity, and directness as they make the transition from childhood to adolescence. As they move into the mid-adolescent range, teens increasingly need discussion and the opportunity to have a say in the design of the structure and norms of the group. Older adolescents need to talk about the future and their concerns about it. Young adults are often more concerned about the present and dealing with life as an adult. Again, homogeneous age groupings are generally more effective.

Unlike an experimental animal that can be raised in isolation in a laboratory, the human animal lives in relationship to others. Therefore, issues of social development intertwine with all those already presented.

Social development

In most cultures, adolescence is the most social stage of development, as young people begin to explore the social roles they will enact as adults. Time spent in school constitutes a major portion of the day and week. Although some young people do isolate from others, the tendency is to be with others.

Identity with the peer group becomes very strong in early adolescence, and provides a new foundation for individuation at a more mature level. Social experiences during adolescence lay a foundation for adult relationships as well.

EARLY ADOLESCENCE

Socially, young people beginning their adolescent journey are concerned with peer acceptance and friendship, but don't easily give or acquire acceptance. The "herd mentality" is dominant, and the need to be part of the perceived norm is crucial. A more mature sense of empathy is building as young people learn to care genuinely about each other.

MID-ADOLESCENCE

By this point, young people need and want consistent friends. They develop loyalties and exclusions, and engage in more long-term relationships. "Best friends" tend to last longer than a few weeks, and some evolve into friends for life or into life partners. The concept of relationship begins to broaden as young people use peers to weigh decisions and choices. Within these relationships, young people explore trust, honesty, and reliability.

LATE ADOLESCENCE

By this point, young people generally have friends of both sexes more often, and have learned to give and receive feedback more easily. Plans for career and further education are important; these plans often test relationships as young people make decisions about school or jobs or where they will live. Adult skills of accountability become more important in school and work relationships.

YOUNG ADULT

As they move out of adolescence, young people often move into a narrower social sphere, focusing their attention on their developing family or a small group of friends. Time spent at work replaces time formerly spent at school; yet, the nature of relationships with workmates and colleagues is different from what it was with classmates. There tend to be fewer connections of a more lasting nature, and generally fewer opportunities to move among different social groups. Relationships are less transient and "more mature."

Groups are great training grounds as well as testing grounds for social interaction. Members with limited insight into the effects of their actions on others may get crucial feedback. Opportunities abound for developing social skills, such as having compassion and empathy, giving and receiving constructive criticism, listening without interrupting, and preventing and resolving conflicts. Although homogeneous age groupings still make the most sense, in groups with a wider range of ages, opportunities abound for learning patience and dealing with people at many levels of awareness. These skills are quite useful for members as they become adults pursuing careers.

Summary

Understanding development is a key to providing a meaningful and useful group experience for adolescents. The leader must be able to recognize and track the stages that the group is going through in order to offer both the kinds of activities as well as the type of leadership necessary to support the group's process in appropriate ways.

It is also vital to understand the developmental challenges that group members are facing during their adolescent years, both those that are recapitulations of the challenges of childhood and those that arise as an integral part of adolescence. It is also important to understand the continuum of development during the adolescent years, and to recognize that the needs of 13-year-old group members are different from those of 18-year-old group members.

It is frustrating, at times, to attempt to describe in language, which is linear, a process that is multidimensional and not at all linear. If this chapter were a multimedia piece of performance art, with singers, dancers, and actors performing against a backdrop upon which a film is being projected, while audience members were interacting freely with the performers, perhaps this would more closely represent a developmental perspective of the adolescent group experience.

I have found it invaluable to view this developmental perspective of group work with adolescents within the framework of another theoretical model, The Therapeutic Spiral™ (Hudgins 2002). This is the focus of Chapter 3.

CHAPTER 3

The Therapeutic Spiral™ as a Framework for Working with Adolescent Groups

A major focus of the work in an adolescent group must be on building the capacity for healthy adult functioning. When I was first introduced to the Therapeutic Spiral Model™ (TSM) (Hudgins 2002) some years ago, I was impressed with how well it fitted into my perception of the roles we develop as we reach the milestones of human development. The reader is referred to the referenced material on the TSM for a more indepth presentation of its principles. I will highlight some of them here.

The TSM categorizes internal roles according to the function they serve in organizing the personality. Within TSM's categories of role functions, the one known as *prescriptive roles* has the greatest application in adolescent work. These are roles of healthy functioning that need to be in place before one can safely address trauma material. As I see them, these roles are examples of healthy, developmental milestones for adolescents regardless of trauma history.

Prescriptive roles include both an array of childhood roles whose opportunity for healthy development is revisited by the adolescent as well as those roles developed for the first time during the adolescent period. This distinction (regarding when in time each role usually develops) will be explored as the chapter unfolds.

Working to support the development of this cluster of roles is the main mission of all adolescent groups. Particularly when one works from a strength-based rather than a pathology-based model (building on what is working for the individual rather than focusing on a diagnosis of what is wrong) a framework for building these roles helps ground the process in appropriate meaning (Table 3.1).

Table 3.1 TSM prescriptive roles

Restoration	Observation	Containment
Interpersonal strengths	The Client	Manager of Defenses
Personal strengths	Observing Ego	Containing Double
Transpersonal strengths		Body Double

There are three subcategories within prescriptive roles that are named on the basis of common function. Each provides an arena for framing several adolescent developmental challenges as well as many action exploration opportunities. The subcategories are: *restoration, observation,* and *containment,* with a number of more specific role functions included within each subcategory. Of these, the first is not only the starting point, but may also be the major focus of the work of the adolescent group.

Roles of restoration: connecting to strengths

Restoration is defined as the ability to identify and utilize personal, interpersonal, and transpersonal strengths. In Chapter 2, I framed developmental challenges in terms of these categories. In the TSM the focus becomes the strengths or skills needed to meet these challenges which are at the core of identity development. The basic questions are: "Who am I?" "Who am I in relationship to others?" and "Who am I in relationship to the cosmos?" During adolescence, the middle question comes first.

Interpersonal strengths

As the infant begins life within an interdependent relationship before a sense of self emerges, so too the adolescent moves toward an understanding of self through the vehicle of others. Younger adolescents often operate more from a "herd mentality" than as individuals. Interpersonal relationships create the foundation for personal as well as group functioning. They provide the adolescent with a chance to revisit the earlier challenge of Trust vs. Mistrust (Erikson 1950; see Chapter 2, p.36).

The opportunity to confront this challenge anew within the peer group instead of the family allows new senses of trust, safety, and competence to develop. For the adolescent who has been traumatized as a child – or who may continue to live in an abusive situation – a great deal of time may have to be devoted to recapturing a sense of interpersonal trust to allow the personal to emerge. That then becomes the initial treatment plan.

Interpersonal strengths include the roles and skills that allow a person to connect to others. They also include specific people, living or deceased, whom individuals have in their families, communities, and social groups, and from whom they draw strength or support. The leader(s) and the group intentionally create a culture that allows members to develop interpersonal strength roles, such as the "caring listener," the "thoughtful giver of feedback," or the "empathic friend." At the same time, group members can each become interpersonal strengths for one another.

It is essential for members to have opportunities to articulate and develop interpersonal connections at every group session and continue to develop the skills that support these connections. These connections, in turn, help create the safe container within which members can explore and express their personal strengths.

Personal strengths

Once group leader(s) and members have been successful in creating safe and supportive interpersonal connections, members can more readily claim their individuality. Personal strengths are those skills that we claim as part of who we are and that we can take with us into most any situation and with most any group of people. These strengths become a significant part of the adolescent's identity and tie in with feelings of self-esteem and a sense of belonging.

Many adolescents, when first queried, may find it difficult to name personal strengths. This can be a matter of low self-esteem, or social prohibitions against bragging. Indeed, one of the biggest falsehoods so often passed on to young people is that it is not all right to feel good about who you are and to say it aloud. For whatever reason, many teens may find it easier to identify strengths in others and so may need the mirroring of the group and the leader to claim these strengths fully for themselves. For example, Linda may not recognize her own courage, but can recognize this strength in Bob. Bob, in turn, supports Linda by reflecting back the courage he sees in her.

Building strengths and helping adolescents identify and connect to them is a vital component of the adolescent group. For many young people (whose experience does not include supportive family, community, educational or work experiences) the group may be the only place in which this opportunity exists.

Connecting to strengths during adolescence does not stop with the interpersonal and personal, however. Young people also need the opportunity to explore and embrace connections to those elements that are greater than self, i.e. the transpersonal.

Transpersonal strengths

Transpersonal strengths are defined as those skills that help establish and maintain a connection to something viewed as "greater than self." Words like "religion," "spirituality," and "cultural heritage" may be used in describing the way the transpersonal is manifest for an individual. It is during adolescence that the individual is drawn to make meaning from life and begins to explore and articulate a newly evolving and more mature sense of the transpersonal. In western cultures, in which rituals of passage and initiation may have come to have less meaning, there may be a transpersonal void that young people seek to fill.

Those who have been raised in a particular faith may reject it or embrace it with a new level of maturity. Young people may try on agnosticism or atheism as they try to develop a cosmology that makes sense. Some may explore various forms of paganism. Others may be drawn more deeply to their own cultural heritage or decide to explore the traditions of the indigenous culture of their region.

Unless provided through a particular religious or spiritual organization, good therapy should be nonsectarian. However, that does not mean that it should ignore the transpersonal. When young people have no outlet for transpersonal exploration, they may turn to substances and other high-risk behavior to fill the void. Gang initiations, accepting dares, and even early onset of sexual activity take on a different meaning when seen through this lens.

For many adolescents, particularly those who are younger or less mature, much of the work of the group may be in developing personal, interpersonal, and transpersonal strengths. With short-term or open groups, techniques that focus on developing and supporting these strengths can employ action structures that can be accomplished within short time periods and that do not necessarily rely on the continuity developed in long-term or closed groups. In Chapter 7, a range of activities will be suggested for developing personal, interpersonal, and transpersonal strengths in adolescent groups.

Once the development of these skills has been addressed, or is at least in process, the next category suggested by TSM upon which to focus the group's efforts is that of observation.

Roles of observation: engaging and disengaging appropriately

Within the subcategory that TSM calls Observation, are the *Client* and the *Observing Ego* roles. Both involve ways of encountering the world and gathering information. The first of these role functions is a continuation of a childhood role that will hopefully express itself in more mature ways during adolescence. The second relates to developmental challenges that are encountered for the first time during adolescence.

The Client

The Client role is the part of self that observes and learns by engaging in action and experiencing fully: physically, emotionally, and mentally. It is the part that chooses to participate in the group and that, once there, engages in action and makes use of the group for personal growth and healing. Healthy children tend to engage fully. Healthy adolescents tend to renegotiate their degree of engagement with their family, friends, and community. One irony of the apparent egocentricity of adolescence is that what may seem to be self-centeredness often comes from a place of uncertainty and arises from "black or white" thinking: either I am everything or I am nothing.

By making the process of engagement a conscious act, adolescents can begin to see the shades of gray that are part of a more mature reality. They can put themselves forward and claim their right to attention while recognizing that others have a similar right. Through receiving and giving attention, young people learn roles of positive interaction in support of others as well as positive action in service of self. They learn to realize: "You are worth my attention and I am worth yours. We can step into action with mutual support and gain control over our lives." Jumping into action, or refusing to, is second nature to the adolescent. The Client helps to bring intentionality to the act.

Not all learning comes from jumping in or refusing to engage. During adolescence young people can also learn to remain connected to the events of the moment while stepping back into a more reflective mode of observation.

The Observing Ego

The Observing Ego (OE) is the part of self that observes and learns by witnessing from outside the action, without judging, shaming or blaming. A major challenge for the adolescent is to develop the part of self that can step back and take a look at what is going on "more objectively." This skill develops over time. It allows young people to begin to evaluate the positive and negative aspects of potential choices without getting stuck in the "shoulds" and "ought tos" or the "goods/bads" or "rights/wrongs," regardless of whether the internalized values that provide these labels belong to the family system or to the peer group.

Being able to move into the witness role, as the Observing Ego, without a call for shame or blame, supports adolescents in learning to think for themselves. The ability to move out of affect and into a more rational place allows the adult skills of problem solving, anger management, conflict resolution, and decision making to develop.

During adolescence, the part of the brain responsible for affection, emotions, and relationships (the limbic or midbrain region) operates in overdrive, making the emotional components of behavior work in high gear. Concurrently, the part responsible for the rational processes of planning, reasoning, language, and development of life constructs (the neocortex) is undergoing a surge of renewed development. The Client helps move the individual into a context in which this significant stage of neuro-physiological development can be supported. As the neocortex develops and is modified, the Observing Ego can grow. Practice in the OE role, in turn, supports the maturation of the neocortex. The process is beautifully interdependent.

It is during adolescence that the ability to witness without judging develops in the "healthy" individual. In the traumatized individual, one who has not developed the necessary foundation of strengths, the development of the nonjudgmental witness is thwarted. Groups may have members who have a trauma history, and leaders may notice that these members are hypercritical of self and/or others and tend to make strong value judgments about issues that others would consider matters of opinion. These are indicators that work needs to be done to develop the Observing Ego function.

As group members are ready and able to work from the perspectives of the engaged Client and the nonjudging Observing Ego, these perspectives can be incorporated into any and all group work. When the affect is flat, the engaged Client helps reconnect group members to their feelings. When it is too agitated, the Observing Ego helps to cool things down. In Chapter 7, a range of activities is suggested for working with the development and support of roles of observation in adolescent groups. Another dimension of working productively with affect fits into the TSM category called containment.

Roles of containment: dealing with affect productively

Containment concerns the ability to be conscious and present, physically and mentally, during times of strong affect, without being overwhelmed. Strong affect is part of the adolescent experience and is connected to increased neural activity in the midbrain (the limbic system), as was discussed in the previous section.

Particularly for those adolescents who have a history of sexual or physical abuse, affect may seem incredibly overwhelming. I have heard group members say, "I am afraid if I allow myself to have that feeling it will take over," or "If I allow myself to feel that anger I could hurt somebody."

Adolescence is a time during which we may learn healthy and effective ways to modulate affect. To support containment, the TSM works with the roles of the *Manager of Defenses*, the *Containing Double* and the *Body Double*.

Manager of Defenses

One way that we learn to cope with intense feelings and situations is through the deployment of various defense mechanisms, such as denial, rationalizing, or joking to name but a few. The process that allows previously unconscious defensive reactions to come under conscious scrutiny, and perhaps influence, cannot occur until the individual reaches a certain level of ability for abstract thought. Therefore, making friends with one's Manager of Defenses is a developmental task of adolescence. This is the part of self that helps us become more aware of our own defensive structures and how we employ them.

It is important to remember that defenses develop for reasons of survival. The goal is not to snatch them away prematurely. Rather, as individuals develop more conscious relationships with their Manager of Defenses, defensive reactions begin to move along a continuum toward greater awareness.

STEP ONE

Defensive reactions, which are at first unconscious and automatic, can begin to become noticed after they happen, or even as they are happening. They are still automatic, but are becoming more conscious.

STEP TWO

As awareness develops, the individual may still employ a defense, but has some choice in the matter. She or he may opt for using a defense as the best tactic available in the moment, but the choice is becoming conscious.

STEP THREE

As the work continues, the individual may move to the point of being consciously aware of a triggering situation, and choose, instead, a healthy response. At this point the TSM would propose that the Manager of Defenses has been transformed into the *Manager of Healthy Functioning*.

In utilizing this construct with an adolescent group it is important to realize that there may be defenses that are important for the group members to keep in place, so the focus is more on the process of choice than on what is being chosen. There are times, however, during which feelings may be so strong and overwhelming that even simple defenses cannot adequately serve to lessen the perceived distress. In these cases, the TSM offers the versatile and invaluable roles of the Containing Double and Body Double.

Containing Double

In classical psychodrama the double is an auxiliary who shares the role of self with the protagonist and offers support, speaks what has been unspoken, or helps to intensify affect. In TSM the Containing Double generally begins with someone holding the role as an auxiliary, and moves toward the role function being taken on internally. The Containing Double's specific role is to help a person contain affect without being overwhelmed by it. This is another developmental skill of adolescence and requires the balance of limbic and cortical functions in the brain. Thus, the Containing Double is also a role that parallels and supports adolescent neural development.

Working with this construct as an intervention provides an understanding that there is a natural, neuro-physiological process in action when one is feeling overwhelmed or experiencing a "flashback." This allows both the group leader and members to demystify as well as depathologize the experience.

Containment is not about the ability to stuff feelings or hold them in, or even to set them aside. It is about being able to create a container large enough and safe enough to hold the feelings without the individual's being overwhelmed. Of all the structures and strategies developed by the Therapeutic Spiral^{TM} (Hudgins 2002), the Containing Double, along with its cousin, the Body Double, have been shown to have great versatility of application and usefulness. Much information about these interventions and research documenting their effectiveness can be found at the Therapeutic Spiral^{TM} website www.therapeuticspiral.org (2005).

The Containing Double utilizes coaching from another or (eventually) self-talk to acknowledge and label feelings accurately, ground the person in the safety of the present moment, and connect them to strengths that support them in containing the affect rather than being overwhelmed by it. When the Containing Double has been successfully internalized, instead of dissociating, leaving the room, or activating defense mechanisms, the person can remain present with the feelings.

Body Double

Trauma survivors are often disconnected from their bodies and bodily sensation. The role of the Body Double is to help bring awareness back into the body. In TSM, this role is taught separately, albeit as a relative of the Containing Double. In working with adolescents, I have found using the two as distinct roles is generally confusing and so teach them as a single intervention. The interested reader is again directed to the Therapeutic Spiral™ website for additional information on the Body Double.

Chapter 7 provides specific strategies for teaching these interventions for developing the capacity to contain affect. Some additional theoretical understanding, more easily understood in the context of the intervention itself, will be presented at that time.

Summary

These presented concepts of the Therapeutic Spiral Model™ provide a useful and user-friendly frame within which group leaders may employ action strategies to build strengths and support the attainment of adolescent developmental milestones. These strategies can also be used to provide a corrective experience for earlier milestones that group members may have missed. As group members develop skills of being able to be connected to their strengths, engage as well as distance without disconnecting, and contain appropriately, many action strategies can be employed to work with the day-to-day issues the members bring to the group. At the same time, as they address their issues, the group members continue to develop their prescriptive roles.

In Part II of this book I offer a range of action approaches for addressing the developmental needs of the group and its members, both in general and in relationship to the TSM. First, as a conclusion to Part I, Chapter 4 addresses issues of leadership and the importance of group norms.

Leadership
and Group Norms

In Chapters 1, 2, and 3, I presented the philosophical and theoretical underpinnings of my work with adolescent groups. To complete the laying of the foundation upon which I built Part II, which explores action techniques that can be employed at various stages of group development, it is necessary to examine two final structural elements of group work: leadership and group norms.

The role of the leader(s)

In the previous chapters, I make reference from time to time to the role of the group leader(s) in supporting the group through its development. I also refer to the different role functions of the leader as compared to the group member. This section begins by exploring leadership in greater depth.

Recipe for leadership

In the early days of my work as an adolescent group therapist, I had the good fortune to be supported by an outstanding clinical supervisor, Michael Conforti, PhD, a Jungian analyst and instructor from my days as a graduate student. As an instructor, Dr. Conforti had a gift for inspiring me to reach beneath the surface and explore deeper levels of meaning. When he was my supervisor, I put this gift to good use.

One day, as we were discussing the importance of the leader's creating a "safe container" for the group, Dr. Conforti and I developed a metaphor for the changing nature of this container that the therapist must provide. In honor of our shared Italian heritage (and in service to my penchant for alliteration), we called it the "Cossa/Conforti Colander Corollary for Clinical Containment" (although he may remember it as the Conforti/Cossa Corollary).

Being a group leader is a lot like making pasta, we mused. In the early stages, good cooks (leaders) put a lid on the pot, providing a secure and closed container, within which the water can come to a rolling boil. When we are ready to add the pasta, however, we take off the lid, allowing steam to escape, so that the contents can cook without boiling over.

Once the pasta is cooked to taste (al dente, of course), we relinquish the pot and pour the contents into a colander. This container holds the pasta in, but allows that which is not necessary to be washed away. Finally, as we are ready to make our meal, the pasta goes onto a plate. At this point, the focus is on the meal, and the container is barely noticed. Not only are group leaders "good-enough" parents, we are "good-enough" cooks.

Co-leading/team leading

Most groups that I have worked with over the years have utilized a co-leader pair. Some groups worked with a leadership team. In running action groups for young people, it is almost foolhardy (although in some settings, perhaps unavoidable) to lead a group solo.

Peter Felix Kellerman (1990) describes the four functions of a psychodrama director/group leader, which I believe hold true in any action therapy: *producer, analyst, therapist,* and *sociometrist*. As I have come to understand these functions: the producer facilitates and shapes the action and keeps the "drama" in psychodrama or drama therapy; the analyst creates and tests action hypotheses and grounds the action in sound theory; the therapist maintains the caring relationship and offers unconditional, positive regard; the sociometrist pays attention to the relationships within the group.

All of these functions need to be operational for good leadership, and it is extremely difficult for one person to perform all of these functions within a group meeting. It is particularly difficult to function as producer and sociometrist simultaneously, so a pair or team of leaders helps assure that the group and its members are being served adequately and appropriately.

PARALLEL PROCESS

It is worth noting that the leadership pair or team traverses a parallel developmental process to that of the group; leaders must realize that issues which manifest in the group may be a reflection of issues existing between or among leaders, and vice versa. Group work-inspired transference and countertransference are important to watch for and manage effectively between the co-leading pair or among the group leaders, and within the group.

As a beginning group therapist I experienced a situation that well illustrates this point. There were two members, I'll call them Rhett and Scarlet, who had met during the group interview, had started dating, and had broken up all before the first official group session. Tension between them often interrupted the process of the group. My co-leader and I tried to address the issue in the group, but with little success. Rhett was unable to talk to Scarlet; rather, he talked about her. Each of them was connected to the group as a whole, but not to each other.

At about this time, my co-leader and I, who had each been experiencing some unexpressed difficulty in working with the other, dedicated a supervision session to our co-leadership relationship. We were able to work through a significant obstacle and were both happy to have made the step, and ready to move forward. At the very next session, the relationship between Rhett and Scarlet seemed also to take a positive turn. The tension between them simply dissipated, and their relationship within the group became productive. At a later point in time, when a life event outside of the group created a new conflict between these two members, Rhett was able to talk directly to Scarlet about it, and they were able to work things through to resolution with the support of the group and the leaders.

"DOODAH" MANAGEMENT

In working with leadership teams, it is essential to be able to deal openly and honestly with those personal issues that are restimulated by the work and which prevent leaders from being clear with one another. In the Therapeutic Spiral Model™ (Hudgins 2002), these issues are given the purposefully nonclinical name of "doodahs." The use of this word demystifies and depathologizes the process, thereby allowing the team to celebrate these potential causes for conflict as intrinsically human and a natural part of team development. Although I may be reluctant to face "countertransferences," "doodahs" seem manageable.

SUPERVISION

Good supervision is invaluable to leaders' clarity and the clinically appropriate functioning of a group. As was illustrated in the example of parallel process above, having someone who is outside the action of the group allows the process and issues to be viewed from a more "objective" perspective.

During years of working with a team, comprised of other staff and graduate interns, I found weekly team supervision sessions a responsible way to support the leaders of various groups, as well as to provide a rich learning environment for interns. Additionally, I received regular supervision, individually or with my assistant program director, to have support for our issues as clinicians as well as supervisors.

In addition to choosing to participate in supervision in order to be clinically responsible, taking part in supervision provides an opportunity for leaders to take legal responsibility as well. As leaders discuss complex clinical issues in supervision, significant aspects are notated in case files and/or group logs to document the therapist's process.

I also feel it essential to the maintenance of confidentiality and informed consent that information of the supervisory process be communicated with group members. Conscientious leaders are not only responsible for enforcing group norms; they are also bound to abide by them.

The importance of group norms

Clearly articulated and consistently enforced group norms are essential to any group, but are especially so for an adolescent group's development. Although the difference between the words "ground rules" and "group norms" may seem semantic, the first implies an external locus of control: these are the rules, and if you don't obey them, you're in trouble. The second is a more organic, collaborative approach: we have come to an agreement on the "normal" way we agree to behave with each other, and we will support each other in remembering to act this way.

Although the *norming* stage of a group is often presented as a separate stage of group development, it is actually an intrinsic part of the forming or beginning stage, and helps create the safety within which group cohesion can develop. If not attended to, and if not formed intentionally and positively from the start, the group will then develop a set of "unspoken norms" which are often very difficult to change.

In the ideal group, if ever there could be such a thing, the norms would evolve from group consensus, and all members would agree to their importance and validity and have a vested interest in maintaining them. The greater the degree of involvement of the members with articulating the group norms, the more firmly and quickly the norms can become part of the group culture. However, in working with young people, some non-negotiable group norms often need to be maintained which, if not spontaneously generated by group members in early sessions, can be set forth by the leaders. In ongoing programs, these norms may have already been voiced, to some extent, by members from previous groups; new members learn that the group and program have a history that predates them, so are generally open to learning what the historical norms have been.

Rather than get caught up in whether or not a particular norm should be included, the focus should be on exploring, in action, how the norms will serve the members and the group in the long run. It is this understanding of how the norms support the work that allows members to accept them, whether or not they have been originally articulated by the current members or revoiced by the leaders. Additional information in Chapter 5 will focus on how to use action techniques to create and understand the importance of norms.

During my tenure at ACTINGOUT (see Introduction), the standard norms fell into the categories of *confidentiality, respect, participation, relationships between members,* and *termination.* Within the first few group sessions, the important aspects were articulated, discussed, and understood, and copies of norms were distributed (see Appendix C). Norms were also revisited from time to time throughout the program year. In the following paragraphs, ACTINGOUT (AO) Group Norms are given in italics, with some accompanying information in regular type.

Confidentiality

Confidentiality is generally among the first norm to be suggested by group members. Taking the time to explore the extent to which confidentiality is upheld, as well as the specific circumstances in which it cannot, helps create a culture of safety that is very important to adolescent group members.

- *All material discussed in the group stays in the group. This applies to group members and group leaders alike.* Although this norm is essential, group members should be reminded that it takes time to integrate, and leaders can discourage the sharing of deeply personal material before the group has had a chance to develop a sense of cohesion. Leaders should also explain the extent to which they discuss group members' material in supervision, in what manner, and with whom.

- *Group leaders are required by law to report cases of suspected physical and sexual abuse, and serious intention to injure self or others. If reporting is necessary, group leaders will work with the member to decide how to proceed.* Particularly in the area of "age of consent" for sexual involvement, many examples can be offered as this norm is discussed and questions may be encouraged to make these reporting requirements understood, both to parents in general information sessions, and to group members in group sessions.

- *Group leaders do not initiate communication about a group member with parents, school officials, or anyone outside the group except at the request, and if possible, in the presence, of a group member.* This norm is the exception, rather than the rule, for most adolescent programs in the northeastern United States and, I suspect, in most places. Feedback from numerous group members has been that this policy is one reason group members quickly feel safe enough to discuss personal material with candor.

- *If group leaders are contacted by an outside person or agency regarding a member, the content of that communication is shared with the member, privately, and the member will be encouraged to share this information with the group.* This norm should be enforced regardless of the nature of the communication. If a teacher says to a leader "Oh, I hear that Anthony is in your group and really likes it" that information is shared with Anthony. It helps him to know that this norm is taken seriously and that "no secrets" are being held. Leaders should also tell incoming group members any information they may know about them from other sources so that the group members become aware that this information is known by the leaders.

- *Any information brought to group leaders by a member about another member cannot be held in secret from the member by the leaders.* This norm provides a mechanism for one member to seek support in working through an issue with another member, while insuring that no leader is talking with one member about another without that person's being brought into the conversation.

Respect

Respect is another norm that emerges, in some form, from members discussing how they would like the group to operate. Part of our role as adult leaders is to develop language that allows a more mature understanding of the concept to become integrated into the members' thoughts and actions.

- *The group is a safe place to express feelings, thoughts, and ideas. Members respect one another's right to be who they are without fear of ridicule.* Along with this norm is an understanding that it takes time for a group to reach a sufficient level of connection within which it is safe to be fully open. By practicing on issues such as preferences in music groups or movie stars, group members can learn how to operate from a respectful perspective that later allows honest discussions of issues such as sexual orientation, life experiences of abuse, etc.

- *No form of verbal or physical abuse, or threats of violence against another will be permitted at any time.* This norm precludes teasing that uses pejorative language. Leaders can explain that each of us has plenty of opportunity to hear negative things about ourselves, whether intended as fact or in fun. A positive peer culture helps members discover what it is like to be appreciated and valued all the time. Members and leaders may slip up on this norm, and ways can be worked out to remind each other, respectfully, when this occurs. The AO culture included the expression, "TNO," which stands for "That's Not OK." In the early days of the program, members adopted this shorthand of a phrase often used by leaders as a way of reminding each other when they were forgetting about certain norms. One member even drew a cartoon of a police officer with the caption, "TNO in progress; request backup!"

- *Members are encouraged to use physical contact with each other consciously and kindly.* Leaders can explain that they are available to provide a supportive hug or hand on the shoulder if requested or needed, but that they will not initiate this kind of contact without first asking permission. Young people have too many opportunities to be overpowered physically and emotionally by adults, and leaders should be very thoughtful about this matter. Although the use of nonsexual touch in a therapeutic setting is a controversial area (partly because all touch has become potentially sexualized), avoiding the issue does not provide the best environment for adolescents. Rather, leaders and group members can work to create a culture in which touch is respectful of boundaries and is used only in supportive, appropriate, and consensual ways. The culture can support members in knowing that having personal boundaries is a good thing and deserves respect.

- *Excessive profanity is not an acceptable form of group behavior or communication.* A distinction can be made between "street language" that is used in helping to express what one is feeling, and "hurtful language" that is directed against another person. This norm supports young people in making conscious and appropriate (to the situation) language choices, rather than in labeling certain words as "bad."

- *Members will not attend sessions under the influence of alcohol or illegal drugs. State and federal laws have made it illegal for people under the age of 18 to purchase, possess, or use tobacco products. All members, regardless of age, are discouraged from using tobacco products during group activities.* Anyone who arrives at a group meeting "under the influence" should be asked to leave. If members are found to be in possession of illegal substances, including tobacco, the substance should be flushed down the toilet in their presence and in the presence of at least one witness. A positive group culture can support members in living substance-free lives. It does not have to require abstinence from substances outside of group. It is important to foster an environment in which members are free to discuss their substance use honestly.

- *Members of the group will respect the space in which the group interacts, and will observe the rules of those facilities within which we work.* This norm fosters an awareness that different behaviors are appropriate to different spaces and situations; discussion and role play can explore what constitutes respectful behavior in the group space, as compared to at school, the local shopping mall, or other contexts.

Participation

From the field of adventure-based counseling, as developed by Project Adventure, Inc., comes the phrase "challenge by choice" (Rohnke 1989, p.5). This is at the core of a philosophy of participation, in which members are invited, rather than commanded, to be as fully involved as possible.

- *Each member is encouraged to participate in all activities of the group. The choice to do so remains the member's.* Group members should be encouraged to be thoughtful of personal energy and wellness of the moment in participating in activities. Leaders may invite participation several times, to support members through an initial fear or block, but the final choice is theirs.

- *Members are encouraged to reveal personal material to the group when they choose, and to the extent that this is appropriate to their needs.* Sometimes the development of appropriate boundaries takes precedence over disclosure and, often, premature disclosure to a group not ready to handle more intimate or painful material can be counterproductive. This norm supports a culture in which each person's material is their own, to share or not, with a sense of timing that serves them, and with guidance by leaders that preserves the success of the group and each member's participation.

- *Success of the program and its benefits to members depends on each member's full, regular, and punctual participation.* Group members should be expected to participate regularly and punctually. Leaders should keep their commitment to punctual beginnings and endings of group meetings as well. Parents can also be asked to sign a statement, as part of the original consent forms, which state that they will not withhold permission for their child to attend a group as punishment for behaviors at home or school. Furthermore, members and parents should be told that information about a member's attendance is not considered confidential information. Parents can be informed if members are frequently tardy or are missing group meetings. If a parent calls to find out if their child attended a particular meeting, they can be told.

- *Any pattern of absence or tardiness by a member will result in review of their member status by the leaders and the group members.* This was not often an issue in groups I have led, but when it was, candid discussion about how members felt about others being absent or late was important.

- *In the event of illness or emergency, members should notify group leaders as soon as the member is aware of the need to miss a meeting. Messages may be sent through other members, if necessary.* If a member misses two successive meetings without contact, a leader may call to check. This policy can be announced to parents and members at initial information sessions.

Relationships between members

This is an area in which there is invariably confusion between recommendations and rules, and which often requires clarification. The clarity more often comes as a result of members' straying outside the norm and then dealing with the consequences.

- *Members are strongly discouraged from becoming "romantically" involved with each other, both during and outside of group activities.* Having a boyfriend or girlfriend is often a priority for teens. The kind of intimacy generated in a group often leads two members to begin a relationship outside of group. Members should be encouraged to consider that, while it can work for two group members to be in a relationship and still be good group members, it is usually extremely difficult for two members to end a relationship and still both remain in the group. This is often a recurring issue in adolescent groups.

- *The group is not an appropriate place for "dating" behaviors.* Although appropriate touch should be encouraged, and physical intimacy should in no way be demeaned or debased, members should be expected to behave in groups in ways that allow each member to be available to all other members. Dating behaviors, cuddling, kissing, etc. separate the dating pair from the group, and so are considered counterproductive and inappropriate within the group setting.

- *Members pursuing friendships with other members outside the group will keep the confidentiality norm in mind at all times.* Unlike the norm for some group situations, this norm encourages members to maintain supportive friendships outside the group, but reminds them that it is often difficult to remember if a particular piece of information was heard in a group (and therefore must be kept confidential) or on the school bus (and therefore is available for casual sharing, i.e. gossip). Leaders, therefore, can recommend that members with multiple relationships with other members try to hold all information that belongs to another as confidential. In that way, a member is not likely to break confidentiality.

- *Members are reminded that paired relationships may limit their capacities to be fully and equally present for all members of the group.* Special and close friendships within the group can be equally as separating as dating relationships, and members can be asked to keep their attention available to all members of the group and to be aware of the tendency to form cliques or special pairings.

Termination

Issues of termination are part of any group from the first session, even if members and leaders assume that all participants will make it to the final meeting. Clarity about expectations around procedures for leaving or behaviors for which someone may be asked to leave is important in creating safety.

- *Leaders reserve the right to ask a member to leave the group, for a session or permanently, if he or she: does not follow these established norms; does not maintain regular attendance; and/or causes severe disruption to the group.* Although members can be encouraged to take ownership of the group, it is important for them to know that the role of the leader is different from the role of a member: the leaders will not shirk their responsibility for maintaining safety and respect in the group.

- *No one will be asked to leave without having the opportunity to have a discussion with the leaders and the group about this request.* Teens have enough occasions to be confronted by arbitrary authority. If someone is being asked to leave a group, they should have a chance to understand the reasons. In my experience as an adolescent group therapist there was only one occasion in which two members were asked to leave, and this occurred only after a number of attempts to support their continued participation had failed.

- *Should a member consider withdrawing from the program at any time, they are requested to discuss their concerns, and/or to say goodbyes with the leaders and the group.* Although not all members will follow through on this norm, the opportunity for closure allows the group to move on with fewer feelings of abandonment or guilt. It may be a difficult time, but it is generally a rich learning and growing experience.

Summary

Group leader(s) must provide a clear and appropriate "container" within which the adolescent group can flourish. Good communication between leaders as well as good supervision for leaders is essential to the process. Clearly articulated and consistently enforced group norms are equally important to the success of the group.

Among the other ingredients for successful action groups are: having a sound theoretical and philosophical foundation for group work; being clear about the efficacy and practice of action methods; and utilizing awareness of individual and group developmental stages to inform the work.

PART II

Action: Utilizing Action Techniques at Various Stages of Group Development

Part I provided a philosophical and theoretical basis for utilizing action techniques with adolescent groups. It reviewed parallels between individual and group development, examined the developmental challenges of adolescence, offered elements of the Therapeutic Spiral Model™ (Hudgins 2002) as a framework within which to work with developmental challenges, and explored principles of group leadership as well as the importance of group norms.

The chapters in Part II explore, in depth, the various stages of group development (Chapter 5: *beginning stage*; Chapter 6: *transition stage*; Chapter 7: *working stage*; Chapter 8: *termination stage*) and the kinds of action activities and interventions that are appropriate to the adolescent group at each stage. Additional material and suggestions for activities relevant to these chapters will be found in Appendices A to D.

Some of the outlined activities presented here are ones I have created and developed in my work with adolescents. Some come from other sources and will be so noted. There will also be some that are a blending of ideas from various sources, or activities that were learned at a workshop or training in the past, whose source I cannot now specify. Some are so widely used by so many group workers that it is hard to know where they originated. While the intention is to credit everything appropriately, apologies if some credits were inadvertently missed.

ACTINGOUT™ (AO) is frequently offered as a model, as I utilize specific examples and insights gained from the 14 years during which I directed this program. It is important for the reader to consider that AO was a community-based, after-school/evening, voluntary, long-term group program that generally accepted new members only once a year. Other settings and situations would need to modify some of the presented suggestions, but the basic principles and activities are applicable across a wide range of group formats.

CHAPTER 5

Action Techniques
for the Beginning Stage

There is an old adage that states: "You never get a second chance to make a first impression." This is certainly true with adolescent groups, especially those for which participation is voluntary. Potential participants must decide if the group will be a safe place as well as whether or not it will offer something of value. The adolescent participant is also checking out whether or not the group will be a "cool" place to be.

Initial contact with group members

The beginning stage of group development starts with the first contact with the potential group member, whether by phone, flyer, or personal presentation. For groups utilizing action approaches, it is important that this focus on action be clear from the start. The idea of action may attract some and scare others away, but providing information for informed choice is essential for laying a foundation of trust. It is also important to indicate to potential members whether or not any previous experience with action techniques is required.

In designing flyers and printed matter about groups, consider whether the flyer is for referral sources, parents, or potential youth participants, and design accordingly. Teen advice can be helpful at this point, since adults often have a very skewed sense of what teens will see as "cool."

The information session

In the ACTINGOUT™ (AO) program, the first in-person contact with potential group members was at an "information session" to which potential members were invited with their parents. Although this practice was not the norm for elective programs for teens in southwestern New Hampshire, it served AO very well. It was made clear that attendance at this session did not commit anyone to participation, but would provide as clear an idea as possible of what the program was and was not.

Since most participants were under 18, parental consent was required. The AO policy was that leaders did not maintain regular contact with parents/guardians. It was important, therefore, for parents to have an opportunity to ask whatever questions they had at the outset. A primary focus of the evening, for parents, was on information.

Because potential members were "checking out" the group, the sessions were conducted *in action* as much as possible. This helped keep everyone's interest level higher, as well as provide the clearest information on what the groups would actually be like. All in all, the sessions demonstrated the basis of "informed consent" both in word and in action.

OPENING CIRCLE

The Opening Circle, adapted from practices developed within the Re-evaluation Co-Counseling community (Jackins 1966), is an opportunity for each person present in the group to be seen and heard, briefly, and to connect to the group in the present moment. Each person is asked to say his or her name and to give an additional piece of information: what town they live in, a recent movie or book that they enjoyed, a favorite food, etc. The specific criterion is not as important as the fact that it is general and not intrusive. The activity is a way to begin building a sense of interpersonal comfort. If people are not ready when their turn comes, they can pass and take a turn later. In this activity, everyone gets to participate in as easy and simple a manner as possible. Although it is true that, for some people who may suffer from extreme shyness or perhaps have speech or language problems, even an activity like this one may be a challenge, it is usually a surmountable challenge.

The Opening Circle is generally followed by a short talk given by the leader(s) that briefly describes the logistics/general information about the program: day and time of meeting, overview of yearly schedule, etc. This is still part of the introductory phase of the meeting, so the leaders purposefully continue to create an environment in which people will feel free to ask questions and discuss issues. Beginning with the most concrete material contributes once again to ease of participation. All the material covered is also distributed as handouts for future reference (see Appendix A for sample handout information). At each juncture, prior to the next activity, there is a pause for questions and comments.

WARM-UP

The leaders then explain that groups generally have some kind of warm-up activity to get members ready to participate in the action of the day. At this point in the session, it is advisable to use an activity that is relatively nonthreatening and that makes only a small demand on participants. One that works well at this juncture is *Eye Contact – Switch Places*. The instruction is simple:

> Look around the circle, and as you make eye contact with someone, switch places with them, moving slowly and carefully enough that people do not collide. If you elect not to participate, you can keep your eyes focused on the floor.

In addition to being simple, the activity also serves the purpose of changing the seating arrangement. In this case, it separates parent from child, as they usually sit together at first, and this is not the preferred arrangement for a later activity. Also, since the activity has a built-in norm about nonparticipation (just don't make eye contact), people can opt out without embarrassment. Once people have participated once, even by opting out, later participation may seem easier.

At this point in the session, the next section of information is addressed, which includes thoughts on therapy and how it works, the policy about family contact (or the lack thereof), confidentiality and its exceptions, and input from parents/schools, etc. Because the talking parts of the evening are kept in short pieces interspersed with activity, a lot of material can be covered without its becoming tedious.

ACTION

The next segment of the meeting is introduced by information about how drama is used to explore issues, both those held in common by a number of members as well as those specific to individuals. An activity that can be used at this point is the *Kid/Parent Circle*. The group remains seated (a safer posture for many), and leaders demonstrate the process.

The facilitator turns to another staff member on his or her right and assumes the role of a "kid" just as the person on the right assumes the role of a "parent." The "kid" initiates a scene about some issues that occur between kids and parents. The scene is short (about a minute) and need not reach resolution. When time is called, the person who was just a "parent" becomes a "kid," turns to the right to a new "parent" and initiates another scene, and so on around the circle until everyone who would like a turn has had one. Passing (participating by watching rather than speaking) is allowed.

Because family members are no longer sitting together, thanks to the Eye Contact game, the activity does not become a contest or actual dramatic interplay between any particular parent and child. However, many actual issues do arise, even though they are played out with other people than actual family members.

This activity also provides an opportunity to demonstrate the concept of role reversal, because each participant moves from "kid" to "parent" or vice versa at least once, and everyone can watch. Additionally, having people who participate passively (by watching) or actively (by participating) offers immediate demonstrations of the way in which one can gain new insight and information from observing or playing the opposite role back to back with the original role.

The information part of the evening is concluded with a discussion on the intake and selection process, program participation expectations, termination procedures, group norms, cost (there is none), and record keeping (the kinds of data maintained about members). Questions and responses are once again encouraged about all information presented during this meeting, or anything else parents or potential participants may wish to ask.

Leaders will then move the group into another action-based activity, usually a *Sociometric Map*. People stand up and move around, imagining a map of the region on the floor, and placing themselves where they live. This has the practical purpose of giving parents a chance to explore carpool opportunities for arranging rides; it's also an introduction to another type of activity to use during group meetings.

SHARING

The sharing portion of the evening takes place in the *Closing Circle*, similar in function to the Opening Circle. This activity invites each person to be seen and heard again before the group is over. The question might be: "What is one thing about tonight's session that you found interesting?" The question is open ended and does not require participants to admit to liking what they did. Again, the option to pass and speak later is available. The facilitator also lets people know that it is acceptable to have the same answer as another person in the circle.

Potential members are then informed that, if they have become interested in the program, they are invited, without obligation, to attend several introductory group meetings to see if they are ready to make a commitment to the group for the school year. Intake and permission forms are distributed with the explanation that, if a young person decides not to participate, these forms will be destroyed; this practice saves the difficulty of sending forms home at a later date and having them returned. Most parents understand this concept quite readily. Staff are available to answer any questions about the forms, especially the reasoning behind asking parents to agree not to withhold permission to come to group meetings as a consequence for behaviors at home. (Sample intake and permission forms are given in Appendix B.)

If this type of information session is not practical or desired, it remains important for clear information to be provided to participants and parents (if the participants are under age) so that issues of informed consent are addressed. Clear information upfront also minimizes the number of participants who drop out and/or parents who pull their children out of group after a few sessions when they find out what the group is really about. It is also possible that even if these sessions are held, some parents may not be able to attend. In those cases, the written information can be provided and questions answered by phone.

Introductory group sessions

Introductory group sessions allow members to understand more fully, and in advance, the group to which they will be asked to commit (informed consent), and allow entry for the latecomers, who always seem to be referred to the group a week or two after the beginning of the program. However, for many groups, a "trial period" is not possible, and the leader(s) will want to begin to build a sense of group cohesion as soon as the group has started. The knowledge that some participants may opt out after a session or two or that others may come in warrants both that the focus be kept on general issues at first and that the leader(s) should help create boundaries against premature disclosure of more serious personal material.

While the group is in the early stages of development, members are still asking themselves: "Is it safe to be here? Can I trust the other members? Will I get anything out of being part of this group? Can I really be myself in this group?" Individuals must answer these questions to their own satisfaction, but the process through which they discover the answers is interpersonal in nature.

Group norms, clearly articulated and agreed upon by the members, contribute greatly to the safety of the group. However, members must reach a certain level of cohesion with each other before they can engage well in the process of creating norms. General program norms can be delineated by the leader(s) at the outset of a new group, then revisited and expanded upon once the group has begun to form a sense of identity and the committed membership is clear. (See Appendix C for sample group norms, discussed in Chapter 4.)

Getting to know each other

Working in action enhances the process by which members begin to build a sense of group identity and cohesion. A variety of techniques is useful in developing a sense of safe connection. At this stage of the group, Opening Circles generally focus on surface information: where people live, things they like to eat, activities they enjoy, etc. This provides an increasing pool of information for members about each other. Using names at each Opening Circle helps members learn one another's names.

NAME GAMES

There are numerous name games that support the sometimes awkward process of learning names as well as help develop group cohesion. One example is *Group Juggle*. This activity may be utilized in a variety of ways, and yet, it is so simple.

With the group standing in a circle, the leader makes eye contact with someone, says their name, and tosses them a soft object, such as a stuffed animal or rubber chicken. This person in turn picks another member in the circle, makes eye contact, says their name, and tosses the object to them. It is fine to ask for a name, if needed. A pattern is established and practiced for several rounds. Then multiple objects are tossed at the same time.

This activity both helps members learn names as well as starts building a sense of cooperation. Some group members may get involved in throwing wildly, but if the group is challenged to "see how many objects we can use without dropping any," or "see if we can cut 10 seconds off our time," the spirit of competition generally pulls even the more wayward members into focus. If within a few rounds the group is not having success with focusing, however, it is better to end the activity without shaming or blaming and to move on.

Group Juggle may also be used again at later stages of the group's development as a way to show the group how it has coalesced. Improved times and higher numbers of objects the group is able to juggle successfully are concrete ways to demonstrate to the group that it has become more unified, cooperative, communicative, etc. Additionally, discussions that occur after the juggling has been ended and the activity is still "alive" can, with more mature groups capable of abstract conceptual thinking, lead to interesting revelations and observations as to how individuals may handle multiple tasks, what causes stress, the definitions of success/failure (catching vs. not catching, "good throws" vs. "bad throws"), and how members react to the noise, confusion, feeling overwhelmed, humor, speed, getting hit, losing objects, etc., all of which occur during this activity.

Alliteration Circle is another activity that can be employed. The first person says his or her own name, preceded by an adjective that begins with the same letter, like "Jolly Jennifer." The next person repeats the first person's phrase and adds their own, for example, "Jolly Jennifer, Mighty Mark." If the total number of group members is small, each member can add something that they like which also begins with the same letter: "I'm engaging Edmund and I like eggnog." The next person has to remember all of this and then add their own name's sentence. The third person has to remember both of those plus add their own, etc., so small groups are usually required for this not to collapse into confusion. In my experience, if the leader is comfortable with games of this sort (and not necessarily great at them him or herself!), members will engage in and enjoy them.

PAIRED INTRODUCTIONS

Another group-building technique that supports those members who may be a bit shy about speaking in front of the entire group is Paired Introductions. From the relative safety of a pair, partners interview each other and then introduce each other to the rest of the group. The shy member is likely to feel more comfortable both sharing about self with only one other member and sharing with the group about someone other than self. Partners are encouraged to coach each other about significant material so that the pressure to "remember everything" is minimized.

This activity can be expanded in later sessions with different partners and asking members to focus on information not previously shared. As members become more comfortable with each other, the introductions can take the form of a celebrity introduction for an awards show: "And the winner of this year's award for having pets from three different species (a cat, a fish, and a hermit crab) goes to Tammy!" The group then gives Tammy a standing ovation as she moves "on stage" to accept her award and give a brief acceptance speech. This activity helps people get to know each other, as well as provides the opportunity to be "on stage" in front of the entire group in a relatively safe manner.

SOCIOMETRIC ACTIVITIES

There are many sociometric activities that can be employed to help build a sense of group cohesion. One of them is the *Circle of Similarities*. Group members stand in a circle and initially a leader names a specific criterion, for example, having a brother or sister. Any member for whom this criterion is true steps into the circle briefly, then steps back. After a few examples, members are invited to offer criteria that are true for them and discover others in the group for whom the criteria are also true by noticing who steps in for the same criterion.

In another variation, instead of stepping into the circle, each criterion may have a different action, such as: "If dinnertime at your house is noisy and confusing, cover your ears with your hands and shake your head." A similar activity instructs members to move about the room and form clusters with people who share the named criterion, such as shoe color, eye color, or favorite movie star.

Members should be instructed that, even with an activity as simple as this, sharing information is always a choice. Exercising the right not to share information that they are not ready to disclose, for whatever reason, is an example of creating clear boundaries, not of being dishonest.

Spectrograms can be used to indicate one's position along a continuum. At one end of the line is "I absolutely love school," and at the other, "I absolutely hate school." Members place themselves along the line to indicate the position that is true for them, engaging in discussion to distinguish gradations of love and hate. Leaders should be thoughtful about what types of information are explored in this manner, as some differences of opinion can become very heated. Tastes in music, for example, are often very personal to the individual and there can be little tolerance for those with very different tastes. If sequenced properly, members can begin to tolerate differences in each other (taste in music, for example) that at first might lead to arguments.

Employing action techniques as a tool for members to get to know each other is generally livelier and more interesting than sitting in chairs and taking turns talking. Action allows members to move about and remain engaged with each other as they discover that there are things they have in common with other members as well as things that are different. Action also covers a lot of ground fairly quickly. For groups with short sessions or that meet for relatively few meetings, this can be a real advantage.

As members build a sense of cohesion, their ability to work together cooperatively will generally increase. They can then approach tasks such as focusing on group norms and exploring their value to the group.

Norm forming

Once a committed group has been established, the norm guidelines previously stated by leaders can be reviewed and the members are then engaged in adding to and discussing them. For norms to become the "normal way we operate," and not just another term for "rules," members must see the value in them and be engaged in the process of norm creation, or personalization of norms presented by leaders. Action approaches can support this process as well.

Leader-developed norms can be put aside for a moment and group members can brainstorm a list of factors that they feel are important to the smooth and safe functioning of the group. Each element can be written on a card or sticky note. These group-generated norms can then be explored to see if they are also stated in the previously presented norms, if they are better or more clearly stated by the group members, or if they need to be added to the "official" version. Once there is some agreement about the basic norms, the group can explore the finer shades of meaning of each norm in action.

Members may break out into small groups. Each subgroup has the task of creating an illustrative scene or vignette about the norm in action, or the norm being violated. The norm violation vignettes are often the clearest way for members to experience the norm, and the reasons for its existence. Role play about incorrectly applying, not understanding fully, or actually violating a norm also provides members with the opportunity to feel what it is like when a norm is not maintained, and thus possibly develop a sense of ownership of the importance of maintaining that norm.

Developing the beginning stage

Once members are committed and norms have been established and understood, the group is warmed up to the exploration of issues. They may be so warmed up that they want to rush into self-disclosure too quickly. There is a tendency for individuals who have experienced abuse and/or severe family dysfunction to disclose information prematurely, before the group may be ready to hear it or work productively with it. It is important, therefore, to preface the group work on specific issues with the development and maintenance of clear boundaries.

Working with boundaries

Supporting a group in developing clear boundaries should not be rushed. Time spent in this manner will provide dividends for both the future functioning of the group as well as its members. If possible, an entire group session could be devoted to clarifying personal and group boundaries.

OPENING CIRCLE

An Opening Circle for a group session on boundary exploration might be: "Give a definition for the word 'boundary.'" This can lead into a discussion about personal boundaries, and to the idea that having boundaries and asking them to be respected are good things. Other possibilities could be: "Give an example of a time in which you did a good job of maintaining your personal space"; "Name a situation in which you find it difficult to maintain your personal boundaries"; or, "Offer an idea about one way that having clear personal boundaries will help this group." The question can be adapted to the level of maturity of the group members, but should serve to clarify the concept of personal boundaries and their importance.

WARM-UP

An appropriate warm-up activity for clarifying boundaries may begin with people moving about the room randomly, without touching, talking or making eye contact with anyone. In increasing increments, contact is established. Participants are told that if at any point they feel uncomfortable with the activity, they can ask for it to stop, and that at each juncture the full activity will be explained before it is put into action.

So next, participants are given the instruction to make eye contact but still not to touch or talk. They are also continuing to move randomly around the space.

Next, group members are instructed to pair up and stand facing a partner, about ten feet away from each other. The pair decides, now talking, who will be person A or B. This next task will be for person A to walk slowly toward person B, who will say "stop" when their partner reaches a point at which their closeness begins to feel uncomfortable. Person A also has the option to stop if she or he reaches a point of discomfort before being asked to stop. Then, roles are reversed. If time allows, members try the activity with several different partners, and with variations, including having a partner approach from the side or from behind. Some other variations are same gender/opposite gender; similar age/different ages; good friends already/don't know one another so well, etc.

Pairs have a few minutes to discuss their reactions to the activity, and then the whole group enters into discussion, including what it felt like to ask someone to stop, be asked to stop, to do the activity with different gender partners, or to be approached or to approach from different directions. This type of discussion allows members to make meaning from the experience; a process that as adults we may assume is automatic, but is still a growing edge for young people. Exploring personal, physical boundaries is a good beginning for the development of members' understanding of personal, nonphysical boundaries.

Furthermore, this may be the very first time that some members have ever asked someone to honor their personal, physical boundaries and had this request honored or respected. Members who are uncomfortable voicing this request may wait "too long" before asking someone to "stop." Interestingly, some members may ignore the order to "stop," perhaps believing that, with a close friend in the group as their partner, it could be "amusing" to push that boundary. What occurs during this activity is all "grist for the mill" of discussion and should not devolve into blaming or attacking anyone.

Although this is "just a warm-up" activity, be prepared for intense feelings to occur for some members. If they do arise, this occurrence is an opportune moment for the leader to demonstrate setting appropriate group boundaries regarding disclosure, emotional displays, and discussion topics at this stage in the group's development, explaining the reasons for setting the boundaries to the extent that the members may understand them.

ACTION

Following a warm-up such as given earlier, the leader(s) may move into *Three Containers Exercise*, developed by my colleague, Sally Ember, Ed.D. The exercise begins as a graphic arts experience. Not only does creating something concrete (a sculpture, drawing or collage) provide an experience of containment, but the artwork also gives a tangible record to use in future sessions.

The facilitator explains to the group members that they are going to look at the "three containers" in which each of them keeps their "personal material." Here are the descriptions. The first "container" (members may create containers in any shape, size or type) holds the things that people can know about you by looking (hair color, eye color, height), and the things that you are comfortable sharing with just about anyone and that just about anyone would be comfortable to hear (our pets, leisure activities, favorite movies). These are the kinds of things group members have been encouraged to share in early group meetings. These are the obvious, the easily knowable, the completely accessible parts of each member's life and person.

The second "container" holds those things for which you need to develop a certain level of trust with someone before sharing (hopes, fears, personal life experiences). These are the kinds of things members may have begun sharing or are getting ready to share with the group. These are less obvious, take some time or effort to know or share, and aren't accessible so easily.

The third "container" holds your most secret and private thoughts and experiences, those things you may only share with a special few people in your lives, or not at all (fantasies, dreams, deeply personal life experiences – good or bad). Some of these things may be shared, after a time, with the group, or perhaps not. Some may never be shared with anyone, anywhere.

Members then have the opportunity to create these containers in whatever fashion they choose, from the art supplies at hand, in two- or three-dimensional designs. They may put "into" each container some items, symbols, drawings, photos, or words that represent each container's contents. There may also be an interest in each container having successively more difficult public access (locks, bars, hidden doors or openings, required passwords, etc.).

Members are asked to consider, by creating and then determining what goes into each container, the importance for themselves and the group that self-disclosure not be rushed, but rather that the group develops to support someone appropriately when a disclosure is ready to be and is appropriate to be made. They are also encouraged, by taking command of the contents of each container, to set boundaries, limits, and categories for their choices for sharing information about themselves. This activity has been shown to improve members' understanding of and use of personal boundaries in their lives in general, not just within the group.

SHARING

Once the containers have been made, discussion focuses on the reasons that it is important to understand the nature of these containers, rather than talking about what is inside them. Members can share their art work and tell the group information such as: "In order for me to let someone see inside this container, I would have to feel..."; or "There are things in this container I hope I will be able to share with the group"; or, "No one gets into this container without my permission." Members can also be instructed to reverse roles with each container and speak as the container, for example: "I am Dave's third container, and you can see by the big lock I have that the material I hold is very well guarded." During the sharing portion of the activity, interesting (and blame-free, judgment-free) discussions may arise once members realize that the choices each member makes about the types of things (giving no specifics) that "belong" in each container may differ markedly for each member.

The point of this important activity is not to disclose information, but to support appropriate boundaries around disclosure, and establish clear norms about sharing information. Talking about when and whether some experiences will be discussed and with whom is an important intermediate step to understanding and developing appropriate disclosure boundaries. It gives the message that one should consciously decide when and with whom to talk about deeply personal issues.

Exploring personal issues

Both drama therapy and sociodrama techniques can be quite useful as the group begins to get into personal issues. The sequence is often not as linear as presented here, so issue activities and boundary clarification activities may intersperse. One way to begin assembling a possible list of issues to work with is through *nondirected improvisation*, a drama therapy approach.

NONDIRECTED IMPROVISATION

As a warm-up to encountering issues through drama, the leader(s) could use *props in a minute* (as seen on the popular television program "Whose Line is it, Anyway?"), in which an object is placed in the playing space and group members find a way to use it as something other than what it actually is. For example, a cardboard tube can become a telephone, a chainsaw, an academy award. The idea is to see how many changes the members can create in a minute. It is a fast-paced and fun activity that helps to build the energy of the group. It also gets people used to quick changes and spontaneous action.

The props are then put away as the group moves into issue-focused improvisation, which may take many structures or forms. The basic idea is that two people begin a scene that can be about any issue or topic. Once the issue is clear, someone can enter the scene as another character; or freeze the scene, take the place of someone in the action, and change the scene to something else.

A list of the issues raised can be made, perhaps writing them on a blackboard, as the action continues. Discussion can then follow about which of these issues members feel are the most important for them and their peers to examine. Some disclosure may start to happen, but the exploration of issues should begin in a more generic manner at this point in the group. As key issues are identified, the group may then move into sociodramatic exploration of the issues.

EXPLORING ISSUES SOCIODRAMATICALLY

In sociodrama, the focus remains on the issue, and members can bring to their role portrayals their own perceptions and ideas of how the role should be played. For example, to create a sociodrama about conflicts that parents and kids have over curfews, one chair could be set to represent the role of "parent" and one to represent "kid." Group members might warm up to the sociodrama by standing behind or sitting on a particular chair and voicing what they feel are the desires, needs, and feelings of the role the chair represents. All points of view, even contradictory ones, can be voiced, and members are encouraged to try out both roles.

From the "parent" role may come statements such as: "I want to keep my kid safe"; "I want to keep my kid from having fun"; "I want my kid to respect my authority"; or, "I don't like the friends my child is hanging out with." From the "kid" chair may come statements such as: "I want my mother/father to treat me like an adult"; "I want to have more freedom"; "I wish my mother/father would stop trying to run my life"; or, "I need to have more time with my friends."

Group members volunteer to play the two roles for the initial scene. As the drama progresses, new members may step into a role and continue it or change it in some way. Again, members are encouraged to try on both roles, and to try out new ways of interacting from within the roles. This may lead to a sociodrama about all the worst ways you can think of to try to get a curfew extension from a parent, or all the best ways. Discussion allows time for members to voice some of their personal frustrations, as well as to explore tactics for communicating and negotiating with parents.

Another important function served by sociodramatic enactment is that it is a training ground for psychodrama. One challenge for using psychodrama with adolescents is that it is often difficult for young people to let go of their own perceptions of how a role should be played and to become auxiliaries in someone else's drama, focusing on being as the protagonist needs them to be. Sociodrama provides practice in role taking, as well as role reversal (e.g. switching from the role of the kid to the parent), and provides opportunities for group members to practice playing roles from another's point of view. It helps build the skills necessary for competence in psychodrama.

VOTE

In *ACTING OUT: The Workbook* (Cossa *et al.* 1996), an earlier work that focused on strategies for creating and performing issue-oriented, improvisational theatre, the use of the acronym VOTE in training actors was discussed. This framework is also useful for going more deeply into scenes such as these. The V stands for Victory, what the character really wants; the O for Obstacle, that which stands in the way of achieving the victory; the T for Tactics, the methods or behaviors anyone uses in trying to overcome the obstacle; and E for Emotion, how the characters are feeling during the process. By exploring Victories, Obstacles, Tactics, and Emotions in sociodrama, group members continue to make meaning of life experience, and can gain insight into how different tactics not only result in different feelings, but in different outcomes.

Summary

Action structures support the beginning stage of group development by helping to clarify what the group is about, establishing clear norms, developing group cohesion, and creating clear boundaries. Action can be employed from the first information and introductory session forward. Action techniques help members get to know each other and the leaders in a manner that is fun and engaging. When directed appropriately, action methods also provide a structure for identifying issues common to group members while protecting personal material from premature disclosure. Appendix D provides additional activities appropriate for the beginning stage.

As the group reaches higher levels of cohesion and trust and members begin to disclose more personal material, other issues will often begin to emerge. These challenges to authority, intragroup conflicts, and absenteeism mark the group's entrance into the transition stage, discussed in Chapter 6.

Action Techniques
for the Transition Stage

In a chapter I wrote about psychodrama with adolescents for the book, *Psychodrama in the 21st Century* (Cossa 2003), I compared the transition stage of group development to the childhood stage often referred to as "the terrible twos." The comparison is an apt one, both in terms of the underlying motivation for the behavior, as well as for the sense of frustration this stage can generate for the leader. Tuckman and Jensen (1977) referred to this stage of group development as the *storming* phase.

Paradoxically, the "testing" behaviors of group members and their challenging of leadership that emerge at this point are indications that group members have begun to connect on a personal and interpersonal level, and that a basic foundation for trust has been laid. It is at this juncture that the group members, like the two-year-old child, feel safe enough to claim their own space and challenge the "powers that be" to discover if difficult experiences can be contained with respect and fairness. Members are discovering that the group has the potential to offer a new kind of experience, and are reacting to this unfolding discovery, naturally, with both fear and excitement, and perhaps a little disbelief.

As Max Clayton states in his book, *Effective Group Leadership* (1994): "In all group work we experience the fact that learning throws us into the new and that at the same time we want to stick to the old and familiar" (p.15).

Getting unstuck

For some groups, the manner in which transition behaviors are handled leads to the group's becoming totally bogged down in a contest of wills. The aware group leader, however, can use action strategies to good advantage in supporting the group members through this unsettling time. Transition is a time of high energy, and this energy can be redirected in service of the group and its members.

Identifying the problem

Instead of fighting with group members or insisting that they "behave," the leader(s) can call the group's attention to what is going on in a way that neither shames nor blames, but normalizes the process.

OPENING CIRCLE

An Opening Circle question can be posed, such as: "What is one way you react when you are frightened by something?" or "What are some examples in your life of times that you have felt stuck?" As the members begin to focus on the process, they can warm up to the idea of self-examination. This is a relatively new skill for the adolescent, and so should be presented as an opportunity rather than a demand.

NAMING AND CELEBRATING

Not only can the leader(s) neither shame nor blame the group members' behavior at this point, but rather the stage of development that the behaviors signal can be celebrated. As a leader, I have often made a statement such as: "As uncomfortable as fear may be, it serves a purpose. Today we want to celebrate that the group has finally reached the transition stage. Only time will tell if we have what it takes to deal with [dramatic pause] '*Secure Frame Dread*'" (Langs 1981).

I provide a simple description of group process and offer the idea that the safer members begin to feel in a group, the more they begin to realize the potential for "real" feelings and issues to emerge. These issues and feelings can be a little intimidating, I tell them, for most members. I invite members to look at the parallels between the behaviors given in response to the Opening Circle questions and the kinds of behaviors that have been happening in group. I further ask the participants if they are willing to examine the process that the group is going through, so that we can decide if we are ready to face these issues that await us at the "other end" of the transition stage.

When the leader is not fighting with or trying to control them, members are generally ready and willing to respond honestly and move ahead when they are ready. Through appropriate transition stage activities and discussions, members become ready to face their fears and to move through them to arrive at the *working stage*.

ART AS METAPHOR

Another approach that I have employed upon occasion, particularly with groups that had started to move out of the transition stage and then seemed to slip back, is to use a graphic image as a metaphor for the group. Prior to one group meeting, for example, I constructed a poster of a hot air balloon in flight.

After the Opening Circle, I displayed the poster and explained that the balloon represented our group. I gave the members markers and asked them to write within the body of the balloon words or images that represented those things that helped the group remain aloft. Words such as: commitment, confidentiality, love, honesty, etc., were common responses.

I then pointed out the sandbags drawn along the basket of the balloon and explained that, although ballast was necessary to keep the balloon from floating away, there were also times when there was too much ballast and the balloon couldn't get off the ground. I asked them to put some words or images within the sandbags to represent those things that were keeping us from getting off the ground. Words such as: people leaving, arguments, people missing group or being late, etc. were common responses.

In each instance of using this type of activity, the discussion moved quickly into a candid look at what was really going on for people. This in turn led to members beginning to articulate what needed to happen to get past the stuck place.

The key, in every instance, was refraining from blaming and, instead, inviting the members to join in the adventure of exploring what makes a group work and what gets in the way. In this manner, the members could begin looking at their fears as well as interpersonal conflicts that needed to be named and addressed, without fear of attack or feeling shamed.

Working with transition issues

Unfortunately, once the problems and the issues have been identified, they do not magically disappear. They can, however, be worked with once they are in the open. Working with the issues directly provides a far more fertile ground for progress and growth than focusing on the negative behaviors that were masking what was actually going on. Remembering that adolescents are still relatively new to more sophisticated cognitive processes, the thoughtful leader can utilize various action strategies to help connect experience to meaning as members work with the issues of transition behavior. Some suggestions are listed below.

SOCIOMETRIC ACTIVITY

As defined in Chapter 1, sociometric activity both examines connections and relationships within groups and provides opportunities for more mature relationships to develop.

Group sculpture

An object is put in the center of the space to represent the group. Members are asked to arrange themselves in relation to the object to create a sculpture of the group, its members, and their relationships to each other and the group as a whole. From their chosen positions, each member makes a statement about why they have placed themselves where they did. Choices are clarified for the group as well as for the member speaking – another opportunity for making meaning. As members listen to one another's statements, some then decide to reposition themselves, having a new understanding of their own situation vis à vis the others.

This group sculpture can be recreated using objects, drawn on a large piece of paper or a whiteboard, or instant photos may be taken and viewed. Members can then step back and observe from a disengaged position. Sometimes leaders can hold members' positions to allow the member to step into an observing place. The leader can then support the group through a process of self-reflection.

The power of sociometric exploration

A specific and detailed example from an early ACTINGOUT group may be helpful at this point. This group of adolescents was participating in a twice-weekly group experience which combined sociodrama, psychodrama, and other expressive modalities with improvisational, issue-oriented theatre. There were 11 members: six male and five female. Several members had prior relationships, and I had noticed these members' tendency to "cluster." The group was about eight sessions into the process and, although it functioned fairly well, the members' stated perceptions of "how connected they all felt" were not congruent with choices people consistently made around seating and choosing small groups for developing scenes. The group would probably have defined itself as being in the working stage. I felt they were still in the transition stage.

I introduced the possibility of sociometric investigation during the Opening Circle by framing a question concerning relationship to the group: "We've been working together for a few months now. On a scale of one to ten, how close do you feel to the group as a whole?" I then brought up the possibility of using part of this session to look at the group and explore the kinds of relationships that had developed and how they supported or inhibited the work of the group.

Questions arose and were answered about how the exploration would go. I knew that if I had suggested doing it with pencil and paper (one way to explore sociometry) there would have been a rebellion. Adolescents object in principle to pencil and paper in groups such as this; it's too much like school. So I let them know we would explore in action, and explained the process for group sculpture. I told them that this was called an *action sociogram*, because this group liked knowing the names of things we did as well as what the things were about that they were being asked to decide.

There was a little resistance and concerns about the possibility of having to talk about "who I like or don't like and why." Concerns came up about not wanting to hurt anyone's feelings. I let them know that the ultimate choice was theirs. Then I set up a spectrogram: at one end – "I think this exploration would be a great idea," and at the other – "I don't like this idea at all." After members placed themselves along the continuum, those who wished to do so spoke from their positions, talking about the pros and cons of knowing themselves better. We then processed the spectrogram information and decided, unanimously, to conduct the action sociogram.

At that point in time, I would rather have postponed the activity, regardless of how valuable I thought it might be, than impose it on the group. My experience in similar situations had shown that when I allow for expression of questions, concerns, and resistances, and entrust the decision to the group, the group will generally choose to proceed. This is one of the "tests" of leadership that helps move the group through transition behavior.

It has also been my experience that, in action, the incongruity disappears and the group creates a sociogram that is an accurate reflection of the group's process and dynamics. This was certainly the case in this instance; the sculpture revealed a very different picture from what had been voiced earlier. There was a cluster of four members at the center facing each other and touching in various ways. These were the members who had been most outspoken for the idea that "all was well in the group." Five members were scattered around them, facing and leaning in. These were the members who had nodded their assent. Two members were off to one side, facing each other. These were the two "silent members." The visual representation supported the group members taking a more honest look at where they were.

After discussion and processing of that activity, group members were asked to form a new sculpture to reflect the group as they would like it to be. The picture was radically changed to one in which all members were standing in a circle facing each other. The group was then able to discuss what they needed to do to move from the current situation to their ideal. The activity was a turning point for the group, definitively moving it further toward the working stage.

REVIEWING NORMS AND GIVING FEEDBACK

Often, as a companion to sociometric activity, a group can revisit its norms to evaluate how well the members and leaders have been adhering to them. Leaders can model operating from a nonblaming perspective by acknowledging what they feel they could do differently to support the group's process. The group can be asked for feedback on the leadership, and members can ask for feedback from the leaders and from one another.

One way to proceed with a feedback activity is to ask members three questions, as each one's turn comes around.

1.   "Are you open to hearing feedback at this time?"

2.   "If so, what kind of feedback would be most helpful to you?"

3.   "How 'honest' (on a scale of one to ten) do you want the feedback to be?"

Members will generally accept feedback, especially when it is clear that it is all right to decline. By setting parameters and levels of honesty, the members remain in charge of the feedback they receive and can generally integrate it in a useful manner.

SOCIODRAMA

A sociodramatic approach can also be helpful to members in viewing and understanding this stage of group development. It allows the group to "play" with the issues and maintain a degree of detachment, which promote greater honesty.

Vignettes

Leaders may facilitate vignettes (brief dramas) that depict "the worst possible group," and then create one of "the best possible group." The sociodrama can be explored in terms of the roles that emerge, such as: "demanding rebel," "compliant peacemaker," "disconnected clown," etc. The roles can be named and then interviewed. This can provide insight into the purposes that the roles may be trying to serve and allow for more conscious choices about how those purposes might be better served. Members can then explore new roles that may better serve their more positive purposes, such as: the "bold articulator of discomfort," the "cautious explorer," the "thoughtful supporter."

Movement activities

There are times when a great deal can be gained by eliminating words. The group can also explore its struggles through movement, or movement and sound, without using language. They can create the "good group machine" and the "bad group machine" to examine the differences between when the "machine" is running well and when it is not.

They can explore member relationships nonverbally as well. If this type of activity is new for members, providing clear structure, at least initially, will generally lower anxiety and increase spontaneity.

Moving forward

To support an action group of adolescents through the challenges of the transition stage of group development, which, in so many ways, parallels the adolescent experience of the world, leaders must truly learn to be "Chaos Riders" (a term coined by one of my former interns, Amy Williams, MA, ADTR). Although it may be difficult and require a tremendous amount of energy and perseverance, "riding" the chaos is a wiser choice than being buffeted by it.

Somewhere along the way in my training as a psychodramatist, I heard the maxim "There is no such thing as resistance, only inadequate warm-up." Whether this is totally true or not, the leader's abilities to track and direct the warm-up of the group and to guide the group toward productive outcomes are crucial skills, particularly during this time of transition.

From chaos to direction: a dramatic example

There was one group I co-facilitated a number of years ago in which a spontane-ously generated drama therapy activity allowed the leaders to move towards pro-ductive outcomes during the transition stage. On one particular afternoon, the energy of the group was moving in so many different directions that my co-leader and I decided not to try to harness it, but just allow it to take its course. We pulled out costumes, art supplies, makeup, props, and puppets and invited group members to go to the items toward which they felt pulled, and to move freely from one to another as they chose.

Some members started drawing furiously. Some got into costume. Others started playing with the makeup. After a time, one member, whose life story expe-riences could be material enough for several after-school television specials, shouted out, "Let's play house!" So began an activity that lasted for a number of group sessions.

The fact that the group leaders assumed roles and interacted from within them put this activity into the realm of drama therapy. I assumed the role of "Grandpa Guido," who visited the "family" from time to time. My co-leader played the role one day of the "kitchen sink," another of the "eccentric aunt" who had come for a visit. Group members assumed roles that either remained constant throughout our days of "playing house," or changed according to the needs of the members.

It was through this activity that the real issues of the group began to emerge, and the group attained the level of functioning that allowed members to address these real issues. Family dysfunction, substance use and abuse, feelings of disconnection and alienation, all came to the fore. The role development that occurred during this activity demonstrated the ways in which action can support the work of the individual from within a role. This activity also provided insight and support for looking at issues "for real" during subsequent group sessions.

The role development of three members in particular marked the growth these members, as well as the group, experienced as they moved through the transition stage. Two members assumed the roles of a pair of two-year-old family members. The "twins" played the entire scene on their knees, keeping the perspective of two-year-olds, but also reflecting a sense of limited power within the group and within their lives. One took on the role of the "bad twin," a reflection of the tactics employed in life of trying to get some control over an unsettling family situation by acting out. The other became the "good twin," also a reflection of the tactic this group member most often utilized. A turning point for this second member was the moment at which the "good twin" uttered, "I'm tired of being good all the time. I want to be bad!" "Naughty" behaviors then emerged, which, in the follow-up sessions, did not lead this member to take on negative behaviors, but did provide role expansion away from having to be the "perfect child" all the time. Interestingly, as the "good twin" became naughty, the "bad twin" started trying on "good" behaviors.

The third role development in this same activity was that of the member who had suggested the game in the first place. Prior to the game, this member was an isolate and disconnected from the group. During the first session of "playing house," the chosen role was that of the pet monkey belonging to the "teen-aged daughter" (who was struggling with substance use along with her "boyfriend," another group member). During our second session, the "monkey" became the "monkey boy," now a human, but a feral child that "Grandpa Guido" had brought back from his travels. In the third session, his character transformed from a feral human to "the man on the couch," some guy who was living in the house when the family moved in, but who wasn't part of the family. In our final session, the "outsider" became "Grandpa Guido's brother, Luigi," who came to visit the family after many years away.

The gradual transformation from animal to feral human to disconnected human to family member provided this participant with a means to begin trying out how it would be to increase his trust for and membership in the group. He also employed role choices to use his close connection with the leader ("Grandpa Guido") to begin making stronger connections to other group members.

Each of the group members used this activity to explore their issues from within the safety of roles first. Through follow-up discussions and group processing of this activity, the group moved through the chaos of transition into becoming a working group at last, a group in which issues could be claimed and explored.

Summary

As groups move into the transition stage, leaders can become so frustrated or triggered by group members' behaviors, words or withdrawals that they "fight back." The ensuing group sessions become a competition for control and power that no one "wins." As anyone who has opposed a screaming two-year-old knows, trying to outyell them or otherwise overcome them creates a lot of turmoil and little or no success. Unfortunately, there are no magic formulae to call on during the transition stage.

Understanding, allowing, accepting, listening compassionately, providing extra time between events, loving, caring, creating and maintaining appropriate safety and limits: these are the strategies that allow both parents and children to survive and thrive through this phase. When leaders can stay present with the group where it is and provide a vehicle for safe expression of feelings, the group can move forward. As the challenges of this stage are successfully met, the tone of the group will become more focused and cooperative. Disturbances will be less frequent and of lesser intensity. Appendix D provides additional activities appropriate for the transition stage.

Luckily, the "terrible twos" phase doesn't last forever; with healthy children, they move from this defiant, fearful, testing time into one of confident exploration of the world, entering peer group experiences of varying types (like preschool or playgroups, daycare or day camp) with interest and enthusiasm. Groups of teens (or adults, for that matter) who successfully navigate the transition stage move eagerly and productively into the working stage, and remain in that stage (barring unforeseen stressors) until members leave and/or the group approaches its ending.

CHAPTER 7

Action Techniques
for the Working Group

In this chapter, I offer a range of useful examples of action strategies for use with adolescent groups in the working stage. The linear nature of books requires that things be placed in one chapter or another; groups do not always develop in so linear a fashion. Ideas and activities are suggested here that may serve throughout the stages of the group's development. Each one's purpose or goal, however, may be different, depending upon which stage the group is experiencing when the strategy is utilized. Therefore, thoughtfulness should be taken to use these ideas in service of the group's development in balance with service to the member.

Erikson (1950) refers to *Identity vs. Role Confusion* as the dilemma of adolescence. Moreno (1964) contends that what we know as the "self" emerges from the roles we play, rather than the reverse. The adolescent action group is an ideal place, then, within which members may clarify issues of identity through role exploration.

As stated in Part I, adolescence provides a unique opportunity to encounter unmet developmental challenges of childhood with new opportunities for success. Roles that were not developed then have a new chance to emerge. The adolescent revisits the challenges of childhood to do whatever "repair" or "upgrading" is possible and then uses this renewed foundation to negotiate the challenges of the present stage and continue to expand the role repertoire. The working stage of the group provides rich opportunities to work with these issues, and possibly to manage these "upgrades."

In this chapter, I first offer suggestions for activities that address adolescent developmental challenges from the perspective of the Therapeutic Spiral Model™ (TSM) (Hudgins 2002), as was investigated in Chapter 3. I then offer strategies for working with adolescent groups in general on the range of "life" issues that generally are encountered in these groups.

Building personal, interpersonal, and transpersonal strengths

Chapter 3 provided an overview of the TSM concept of restoration, focusing on the building and reinforcing of personal, interpersonal, and transpersonal strengths or skills. In order that group members may develop a cognitive frame for the work, it is important to teach them the language of the theoretical framework employed by the leader(s) and to use it with them. Sometimes words alone cannot convey meaning as well as a simple action strategy. Members can be asked to stand in a circle and place their hands on their chests and say, "Personal." Then hands are extended out to make contact with the person on either side while saying, "Interpersonal." Finally, group members disconnect from each other and point hands upward and give them an "alleluia" wave and say, "Transpersonal."

In my experience of using this technique, members having trouble with the correct word will often communicate with the correct hand gesture instead. Getting the words correct is less important than developing an understanding of the importance of connection to strengths and understanding the relationships among the various kinds of strengths.

Opening and closing rituals

Opening and closing rituals can provide excellent means for articulating and claiming strengths, whether personal, interpersonal, or transpersonal. An action structure used during Therapeutic Spiral™ (Hudgins 2002) weekend workshops is to create a *Circle of Scarves*. Members select from an assortment of colored scarves and indicate which strengths the chosen scarves (and/or colors) represent for them. Members then place their chosen scarves around the room, creating a *circle of safety*. The action of the weekend happens within this circle. The process involves naming and concretizing strengths from any of the categories. Concurrently, members consciously work to create interpersonal safety and cohesion, and also to recognize the potential for these strengths to be present in the work of all members.

For an adolescent group meeting several hours per week, creating a scarf circle of safety before each meeting is not time efficient. However, the function of the activity need not be ignored. Groups that meet regularly, particularly when they have reached the working stage, have the advantage of being able to operate from an already generated sense of cohesion. The ritual, then, does not have to create cohesion, only to connect members to the sense of cohesion they have already created. The activity also gives the members an opportunity to reflect on strengths and roles that are important to them at this point in their growth. If the ritual has once occurred, even though scarves have been put away since then, members may elect to reselect or put their own scarves some place visible to remind themselves of their strengths during any group meeting.

One approach that can be used is to ask members to reflect on a certain type of strength for the evening (e.g. a strength that helps me deal with change) that is selected by leaders during their warm-up prior to the meeting and which is relevant to the group's process. Members then find an object from art supplies or the sand tray area that can represent that strength. After participating in this ritual for a time, members often bring objects with them from home to use as well. These objects may be used in answer to the question of the evening or in naming other strengths the members want to reinforce. Then, standing in a circle, perhaps around a table, the objects are set out and the strengths are named. Once the strengths are named, a candle can be lit in the center of the table to be kept burning until the end of the group session.

The ritual provides the opportunity for personal strengths to be named. Inter-personal connections to group members and to those outside the group who make up important support networks can also be acknowledged. Transpersonal strengths can be named, and the act of creating ritual addresses the need for transpersonal connection in a nonsectarian way. At the close of the group, the members can reflect on how their strengths may have changed during the group, or on new strengths that have emerged. As strengths are internalized, the session ends with the extinguishing of the candle.

Warm-up activities

At some group meetings, the members may be so warmed up by the end of the Opening Circle that they are ready to move into action. Often, they are not, and require some sort of warm-up activity that can help the group look at itself, discover or explore a common issue, or determine who will be the protagonist, if the evening is going to be psychodrama focused. It is up to the leadership team, working with the group, to determine "where they are" and "where they want to get to." The warm-up activity is a step along the path. It serves the practical function of decision making, while enhancing the development of strengths.

Sociometric activity can be well employed as a restorative warm-up. Group sculpture, detailed in Chapter 6, can be a useful tool in aiding the group's explora-tion and understanding of the changing nature of relationships. If the group did a sculpture early in their work together, it will likely be different at this point. Referring to notes, photos or drawings of the group sculpture from an earlier session allows the group to see both where they are now as well as where they were then.

Strength cards

As mentioned earlier, it is not always easy for young people to identify and claim personal strengths. My colleague, Kamala, found an action approach to dealing with this problem. Members of the group are asked to come up with ideas of personal strengths that someone might have and to write them on index cards. The cards are passed around the group and members draw images or designs on the cards to illustrate the concepts in some way. The members are warming up to the idea of personal strengths.

The creation of these cards can lead to further exploration. They can be spread out on the floor and members asked to go stand next to a card that represents a strength that they know they have at least some of. As members look around the group, they discover that, among them, they have a collection of strengths that none of them has alone. Then they are instructed to go stand next to a card that represents a strength they would like to have more of in their lives.

Psychodramatic and sociodramatic vignettes

In continuing to work with the strength cards, members can enter into dialog with each other about how certain strengths have been developed or work for them. A strength can be fleshed out into a role for further exploration. For example, the strength of "courage" can become the "courageous explorer," or the "courageous defender." "Caring" can become both the "caring friend" as well as the "self-nurturer." A sociodramatic vignette can be enacted in which the various roles talk to each other.

Psychodramatic vignettes can be developed in which members role reverse with their known strength to get ideas for how to invite a new or emerging strength into their lives. This can be enacted with three chairs: the center one represents the group member working here today; the two outer chairs represent the developed strength or role and the emerging strength or role. The group member can move among the chairs freely, or select auxiliaries from the group to play the roles and then engage them in role reversal and dialog.

Transpersonal strengths can also be explored through a sociodrama that takes place in "Heaven," on "Mount Olympus," or in the "Realm of the Oversouls." Although care must be taken not to create sectarian disharmony, an opportunity to move into that part of self which is connected to a sense of the transpersonal and, from that role, dialog with others in their corresponding roles, can make the unconscious desire for meaning more conscious and help connect the individual to their "faith" more maturely and strongly.

Collage and artwork

There are times when the expansive nature of drama or movement is contra-indicated with an adolescent group. Members may arrive already hyperactive or overstimulated, or the energy of the group may be low. Artwork can be useful for containing excess energy and connecting a low energy group to themselves and each other. Many adolescents enjoy drawing. Many do not. The opportunity to create collage, using pictures and words cut from magazines, offers even the least "artistic" a means of graphic expression that can be "good enough." A word of warning, though: it is a good idea to have the pictures and words already cut out of the magazines. Otherwise, group members may get more involved in the magazines than in the art project.

Collage/artwork can be used to create "self-portraits" of strengths, joys, and important issues. They can be done on standard paper, or even on the tracing of a person's body done on butcher paper. One variation I have used, particularly with groups that have been working with Drago-Drama (archetypal psychodrama of the "dragons" that keep us from our "jewels of great worth"; Cossa 2002), is to create a *shield of self-confidence*. The shield can be any shape, and contains images of personal, interpersonal, and transpersonal strengths: those things that contribute to our self-confidence.

Group members may continue throughout their time together to work on issues of connecting to and supporting their strengths. Additionally, action strategies can be employed to support the development of roles of observation.

Developing the ability to observe from within and without

As stated in Chapter 3, the TSM observing role known as Client, which manifests in the ability to engage directly in what is going on and learn from it, is one that is already developed in childhood and matures in adolescence. The development of the "dispassionate witness" role, or Observing Ego, is an experience that is part of adolescent development.

In working with these roles, group members learn how to move away from the Client (engaged action) when their perspective is too narrow or when affect becomes overpowering. For many adolescents who participate in psychodrama, watching another's drama can evoke so many feelings from their own material that they may either dissociate or want to physically leave the room. They can learn that there is an alternative action: namely, to move into a more witnessing space, cool down a bit, and remain present. Once the members discover that this movement out of Client role and into Observing Ego role can help them to stay present in the group, they can begin working on ways to use this strategy in affect-laden life situations.

Changing perspectives

One way to introduce these concepts is by a role play activity. The group space is divided into thirds. One portion is the Action space, one the Client space, and one (furthest from the action) the Observing Ego (OE) space. Two team members (if available) engage in a scene in the Action space. If group members are used in this capacity, they should be rotated so that each group member has a turn participating from the Client and OE positions as well. The instructions are given as follows:

> Watch the scene take place in the Action space.
>
> If you are sitting in the Client space, then allow yourself to relate to the scene in multiple ways. See which character you identify with. Imagine what the characters are thinking and feeling. Allow yourself to think about situations in your life that are similar.
>
> If you are sitting in the OE space, try to notice what is happening without judging. Do not interpret what people are feeling and do not try to connect to similar experiences. Merely notice volume of speech, movement on the stage, content that is expressed. Do not judge who is right or wrong, just notice and be able to describe, in nonjudgmental language, what you are seeing.

The scene commences and generally involves some sort of intense conflict. The content should be something with which group members can readily identify. After a time, the scene is paused. People in the Client area are asked to describe their reactions. The following sorts of reflections may come from the Client space: "The mother is trying to control her daughter"; "The mother and daughter are fighting"; "The daughter feels suffocated by the mother's overprotectiveness"; or, "That is so much like what happens between me and my mother."

From the OE space, comments can be (and may require some coaching at first to keep the judgment and affect out): "Each time the mother's voice got louder the daughter's voice got louder as well"; "When the mother moved toward the daughter, the daughter moved away"; "The mother did not want the daughter to go out on a school night"; or, "The daughter said that she was the only one in her class whose mother was so restrictive."

As members get more skilled at making nonjudging comments, statements concerning value can be allowed if they are made without affect. These statements might include: "The characters seemed to care a lot about what was going on"; or, "The characters seemed not to be taking in each other's point of view."

As with any new skill or awareness, the opportunity to practice in situations for which one has little vested interest in the actual outcome allows the skill to develop fully. Then, it is more likely to be employed in actual life situations. Group members can become more conscious of situations in which they can operate most effectively from Client, and when the distance of OE would better serve them.

Role awareness for group meetings

Over time, group members learn to identify which space they are in or need to be in during the group session. During the selection of a protagonist for a drama, members can be asked to put themselves forward as a potential protagonist (Action), to be available to play auxiliary roles (Client), or to be a witness (OE).

One group member, with whom I worked for a number of years and whose tendency was to run out of the room when the action got too intense in a drama, made a tremendous step forward in her work the first time she decided to move back into the OE space instead and to remain present for the drama. In subsequent weeks, she would include in her group check-in comments like "I am ready to really get involved tonight" or "I have been feeling a bit overwhelmed this week. I think I need to be more in the witness space tonight."

The fact that members can begin to make conscious choices and learn to modulate affect in healthy ways are indicators that an important developmental milestone is being reached.

Using the Observing Ego position

During a drama, the protagonist can be brought out into the OE space (traditionally called the *mirror* position in classical psychodrama) not only to cool down affect or help engage a stuck protagonist, but also to notice and observe what is happening in the drama without judging. If the voice of the "Inner Critic" starts to emerge from this space, the director can coach the protagonist to set that voice aside and stay for a moment in the OE Role. The "Inner Critic" is not a role of support and growth, but rather is generally an internalization of external critical voices one has heard throughout life. These voices scold and devalue. By supporting the development of the OE, one can develop an "Inner Evaluator" instead, to offer helpful feedback instead of scolding.

Role reversal

Each time a group member is invited to role reverse with another, whether in a drama or during a group meeting, there is an opportunity to strengthen the OE role. A true role reversal requires the taking on of the perspective of the other without judging. Learning to see things from another's perspective is a key challenge of adolescent development.

eliminated. The important thing is for members to develop the ability to identify their needs (a personal strength) and to ask for support (an interpersonal strength).

Sociodrama

Sociodrama is a good way to explore issues of common concern and for sessions in which there is no clear protagonist. It also provides a way to explore issues that members may be considering bringing to the group as personal concerns but, before owning them, want to see how their fellow participants will react to these issues.

EXPLORING A CENTRAL CONCERN

At any given group session, common issues or themes may be apparent for a number of members, such as the issue of dealing with pressures to become (more) sexually active. A sociodrama can be structured in which members can explore roles of those young people who have decided they are not ready for (more) sexual activity, as well as those who are encouraging them to "have sex." Additional roles might be those who have engaged in intercourse or other intimate sexual activities and are pleased with their decisions, as well as those who are sorry they did not wait a while longer. As the drama progresses, members are encouraged to try on each of the roles and experience the issue from the possible perspectives of each role. They may be surprised with some of the motivations they discover from the various roles.

As members explore various strategies through role, and witness others doing so, their awareness of possible options for encountering the particular situation can grow. Within the sociodrama, a particular member is not necessarily playing himself/herself, and may therefore feel freer to explore the issue in greater depth from the safety of distance or depersonalization.

EXPLORING GROUP DYNAMICS

Group members can also take a look at themselves as a group, through socio-dramatic enactment. If, for example, members' participation covers a wide range of both active involvement and hesitancy to share openly, roles such as the "ever-ready utilizer," the "guarded supporter of others," and the "fearful secret holder" can be enacted. The "concerned facilitator" and the "caring truth-speaker" may also become involved. Members can explore various roles, especially those that are furthest from their own. Roles can be taken to the extreme, as long as this action is not used as a way to make fun of the way another member behaves in group. When the roles are painted in broad strokes, each member is more likely to look at their relationship to these roles than if the roles were created too personally.

Characters can be asked to offer their inner thoughts as *soliloquy*, the speaking aloud of inner thoughts, or members may take turns playing each other's "inner thoughts and feelings." When entered into with a sense of play, the heaviness of the issue drops away, and members are more likely to discover some of the dynamics in which they have been engaged. Members can also gain a great deal from stepping out of role and witnessing the drama from time to time.

BUILDING COMPETENCE FOR PSYCHODRAMA

Sociodramatic enactment also provides good rehearsal for the various skills needed to participate fully in psychodrama. Adolescents need to build their ability to see the world from another's perspective before they can serve as good auxiliaries to each other. Their natural tendency is to play their own perceptions first, which is appropriate to sociodrama. As they gain experience with taking roles that are different from their own, as well as accepting suggestions for other ways to play sociodramatic roles, their ability to role reverse also increases. Working in sociodrama enhances the ability to put oneself in "another's shoes."

Sociodrama: Who's in Your Shoes? by Patricia Sternberg and Antonina Garcia (1994) provides a thorough and detailed description of sociodrama in its various forms.

Psychodrama

As the group develops a good working relationship among members, and as members gain competence in action modalities, psychodrama can be a most powerful and effective tool for working with adolescents. Psychodrama can be either intrapsychic (exploring the protagonist's inner reality), interpersonal (exploring issues of relationship), or scenic (related to specific scenes or events in a person's life.) The following are a few ideas for working with adolescents in each of these areas.

INTRAPSYCHIC PSYCHODRAMA

Adolescents work very well in the arena of intrapsychic psychodrama and, indeed, this type of work is extremely supportive to the adolescent tasks of self-discovery and identity formation. Working with prescriptive roles, described earlier in this chapter, is intrapsychic psychodrama. *Concretizing ambivalence* ("there is one part of me that wants X, but another part of me that wants Y") is another form.

Working with issues of abusive relationships from an intrapsychic rather than interpersonal perspective can help clarify the real issue and help the protagonist get some distance from the personality, charm, or power of the abuser. An intrapsychic drama allows the protagonist to have a conversation with the part of self that really wants to be in a relationship ("I want to have a boy/girlfriend") and the part of self that sees that this particular relationship is hurtful ("I want better for myself than this").

In early stages of group experience with the modality, and with younger members whose ability to remain present for each other may still be developing, it is often a good idea to offer activities in which all who so desire can participate. A series of brief *psychodramatic vignettes* around an intrapsychic theme can be employed to help members warm up to other personal issues that need to be addressed.

One such warm-up was spontaneously generated at a group meeting from a comment of a member during Opening Circle. It is called *Rabbit/Tiger/Dragon*. Three chairs are placed in the playing space representing the three animals. Members spend a few moments in each chair reflecting on how active each of these parts of self may be in the moment. The "Rabbit" represents the part of self that is withdrawn or frightened, the "Tiger" that part that charges boldly ahead but not always with forethought, and the "Dragon" (in an eastern sense) that part of the self that is wise and thoughtful. If used as a warm-up, the members may move fairly quickly from chair to chair and then move into selecting a protagonist to do a bigger piece of work. If the group has decided to share the time, a more indepth approach can be taken, and then the vignettes become the "action" of the group session.

INTERPERSONAL PSYCHODRAMA

Operating effectively within more mature relationships and handling conflict productively are goals of adolescent development as well. Interpersonal dramas allow the protagonist to try out various ways of relating to others. They offer the chance to say things we thought we could not or should not say, or the things we wish we had said, and see where this expressiveness could lead.

The key to successful interpersonal drama is often well-placed role reversal in which the protagonist can develop new insight into the other person from operating sincerely within the role of other. It is important in such a role reversal to coach the protagonist, if needed, to allow this insight to develop rather than just have a demonstration of the protagonist's negative projections of the other. Questions like "What are you really feeling about X?" or "If you were really honest about this, what would you tell me?" can allow the protagonist to take on the role more fully and explore the point of view of the other.

In some instances, the protagonist may just need to vent and express the pent-up and unexpressed feelings without any response. Using an empty chair, an object, or a silent group member may be more appropriate. Especially in cases in which the protagonist is expressing thoughts and feelings toward someone who may have been a perpetrator of abuse or with whom the member is already overidentified, it might be better *not* to have a role reversal. A dressmaker's dummy, dressed as a woman on one side and a man on the other, is quite suitable for these types of scenes. If group members or leaders hold such roles, it is generally a good idea to cover their face with a mask or cover their head with a scarf to symbolize that the words are being directed at the role and not the person.

SCENIC PSYCHODRAMA

There are times when it is worthwhile to revisit a particular scene or event with the protagonist; to do this, it is important to spend some time in setting the scene. This is particularly helpful with protagonists who are slow to warm up to action. Good scene setting can deepen the psychodramatic experience. It can also provide a social context for working with a multiple interpersonal issue (e.g. mom, stepdad, siblings, and stepsiblings).

In addition to role reversing the protagonist with other people in the scene, it can be extremely helpful to role reverse with inanimate objects. This is a great way to support Observing Ego development: noticing from a neutral place. We have heard the expression "If these walls could talk." In psychodrama, they can.

Some years ago, I brought Zerka Moreno to the town in which I was working to offer some special workshops. One was for a group of youth workers, and we had a former member of one of my groups come to be the "adolescent protagonist" for a demonstration drama that Zerka would direct. The young man, just slightly over 18, set the scene involving himself and his employer on the truck that he drove to deliver product. The turning point of the drama was when Zerka directed, "Role reverse with the truck." Suddenly the drama moved beneath the surface and the real issues began to emerge. (Incidentally, that young man went on to become a car salesperson.)

Cautions and complexities in using psychodrama

With adolescents, a certain amount of competency building is required for participants to use the modality of psychodrama well, especially in terms of being able to hold a role as defined by another and in service of the other's perceptions and process. In addition, it is important to remember that psychodrama is a powerful modality for exploring thoughts and feelings; participation in psychodramatic action can bypass members' normal defenses. Participants may move into an intensity of affect beyond that for which they or the leader(s) are prepared.

It is not my intention in this book to try to teach anyone how to be a psychodramatist. There are training programs around the world to serve that broader purpose. However, I hope I have encouraged some to learn more. For a comprehensive and user-friendly introduction to the field, I recommend Blatner (1996, 2000). I trust this book provides some new ideas and perspectives for experienced psychodramatists as well.

Additionally, the principles of working safely with intense trauma material are beyond the scope of this chapter. It requires training and experience to conduct "trauma dramas," and is seldom appropriate in an adolescent group, particularly with younger adolescents. Young teens are generally too close to the traumatic experience; or they may be living in the same family situation in which the trauma occurred or even with the same family members who perpetrated the trauma, and their susceptibility for being retraumatized is too great.

The focus with adolescent groups is generally working to build the prescriptive roles. Unless these are safely in place and well developed, the risk of retraumatizing the participant is very high. That is not to say that adolescent groups do not deal with intense issues, but rather that the focus should more often be on the current situation rather than on revisiting earlier trauma.

Group leaders should also be very cognizant of time issues when working psychodramatically. As a general rule, it will always take longer than you think it will to do a drama. It is also important to have time for *de-roling* and *sharing* at the end of the drama, as well as for *cooling down* and *group closure* before members leave the group space.

De-roling, the process by which members clearly and cleanly let go of roles that they have been playing, is important to do for these reasons: so the members do not take elements of the roles with them; so other members no longer see those elements in those who played the roles.

Full sharing, which is about telling the protagonist how his/her work reminds you of your own issues, allows the group to experience the ways in which the protagonist truly does the work of the group. It also helps members realize that it is possible to get their needs met even if they are not selected to be the protagonist.

A good cool down and group closure allow members to make choices about how emotionally vulnerable they want to be as they leave the group and go on about their lives. (See Appendix D)

Psycho / socio / drama therapy

There are some approaches to working with adolescent groups that move fluidly between psychodrama, sociodrama, and drama therapy, or that may be more of one if conducted one way and more of another if conducted another way. The name we give to the modality really doesn't matter. The key is to work in ways that increase spontaneity and creativity for all concerned.

ROLE TRAINING

Role training has somewhat different definitions depending upon where in the world you have been trained. Which modality name is most appropriate to it is a matter of whether the focus is on the individual or the group, the degree and type of involvement of the director, and the slant or twist that the leaders bring as a reflection of their training. It is used here to include work that can be intrapsychic, interpersonal, or scenic and that involves the development of new roles, support for emerging roles, and rehearsals for pending or potential events. The first two have been covered to a degree in the section on working with prescriptive roles. The third is an area that can offer very practical support to the adolescent group member.

In recent decades, a number of prevention curricula have been developed to work with young people on issues of substance abuse, HIV, pregnancy, and violence prevention. What they all have in common is the opportunity to practice healthy social skills for refusing, negotiating, or resolving. With role training in these areas, not only do youth participants get to practice the healthy behaviors, they also get to experience the consequences of poor choices in *surplus reality* rather than in real life. A young group member with whom I worked once commented, "I have been thinking about trying marijuana this year, but I feel I got enough of the experience of it from doing scenes about it. I've decided it is not for me."

In addition to "prevention" practice sessions, role training can also be used for preparing for a job interview, talking to a teacher about a missed assignment or grade, negotiating with parents about an extended curfew, or letting a special person know how you feel about them. Most people have the experience of rehearsing these kinds of things in their minds, but doing it aloud with a group provides the opportunity for feedback from the group as well as the first-hand experience of the effect that various approaches may have.

ARCHETYPAL DRAMA

Working with myths, legends, fairy tales, folk tales and the like can also provide a rich source of experience for a group. Moving from direct reality into metaphor provides a bit of distance that sometimes allows a more honest look at personal material. It also allows participants with a range of issues, experience, and competence to work together productively with each taking from the experience at their own level of awareness. These kinds of activities are also fun and allow participants and leaders alike an opportunity to tap into their creativity, spontaneity, and sense of play.

Many of the young people I worked with over the years were Live Action Role Players (LARPers) and were accustomed to engaging in action through roles. Over a period of time, I worked with them and with groups of young people and adults around the world to develop *Drago-Drama*, an archetypal quest to confront the dragon and reclaim the "jewel of great worth" (see Cossa 2002 for a full description of this process).

Working with the stories and tales of one's culture also encourages a deeper connection to one's family and traditions. It is another opportunity to nurture the transpersonal growth so important to the adolescent. Working with such material in a multicultural setting also allows a building of interpersonal connection across the cultures as tales and stories are shared and their similarities as well as differences emerge.

WORKING WITH SCRIPTED MATERIAL

There are also times within a group in which working with the reading, acting and/or production of scripted material can greatly support the work of the group and its members. In settings that are more educational or psycho-educational than therapeutic, scripted material allows a level of involvement and personal growth that other types of activities may not. Developing a character and working from it, even when the lines are proscribed by the dialog, also allow individuals the opportunities to have some distance from personal material that may be hard to look at. A role may give an actor the opportunity to explore a personal issue in greater depth. It may also allow the actor to try a new way of relating to others and the environment. Therapeutic role assignment principles suggest that the leader/ director cast the show more from the perspective of how the roles will serve the actors than the reverse.

Summary

Although in many respects the real work of the adolescent group is learning to be a group, when this goal is achieved there is a tremendous amount of exciting territory that can be covered in action. The first step is laying the foundation that allows members to work together well. The next step is creating the safety that allows members to claim and develop all of their potential within the group as they encounter and explore the developmental challenges of their age and stage in life. Appendix D provides examples of additional activities appropriate for the working stage. The variety of ways to utilize action approaches to work with the issues of the moment for group members is bound only by the imagination and spontaneity of the leader.

The final chapter in Part II looks at the issues that arise around termination and how action approaches can support a group in experiencing a "healthy" ending.

CHAPTER 8

Action Techniques
for Termination

Many adolescents have difficulty with endings, particularly if the experience that is about to end has been a positive one. Anyone who has been involved in a high school play will remember the tears that accompany closing night. The same is certainly true with a counseling or therapy group in which members have opened up to themselves and each other. Negative responses to the group's impending end vary widely, but basically fall into two categories: inappropriate, or "dysfunctional"; appropriate, or "functional."

Signs of members' difficulty with termination may manifest in individual or collective ways. Often, as the group reaches the end of its sessions, individual members may increase rates of absenteeism or may even drop out. Members may minimize the importance of the group while still attending the sessions, or get involved in other things that cause them to miss meetings. During group meeting times, some individuals may feel negatively towards other members' lack of attendance, or about their minimizing the importance of the group, and behave or speak negatively towards those members. This can cause factions or cliques to form spontaneously solely based on the ways in which members respond to the group's ending. These and other less-appropriate responses are quite common, so appropriate responses ought to be fostered intentionally for everyone's benefit.

Grief at endings is an appropriate response. Group leaders can support members in expressing this grief. Leaders can also assist members in recognizing the accomplishments of the group and in finding ways to carry these achievements forward in their lives. The close connections formed between members, or between members and leaders, can be appreciated and discussed openly, with positive feedback sessions, validation time for each member, or appreciation exercises of other types. Termination may be painful, but it can also be healthy and productive.

Aware leaders begin doing termination work with the first session, and continue in every session. This work includes setting and maintaining clear boundaries, modeling open communication, fostering group bonding, teaching and practicing the skills involved with being able to face one's inner truths directly (even when these truths show one's pain), and consistently naming "what's really going on" (vs. allowing unconscious displacement to remain unexplored).

Awareness of ending at the group's beginning

It is important that a group begins with its end clearly defined. Even if, for example, there will be the possibility to sign on for another eight weeks once the first eight have been completed, each segment of the group experience should be defined as a distinct entity. Indeed, even if only one member leaves or one new member joins, it is no longer the same group. Learning both that things do end and that life continues are vital lessons for an adolescent. These are lessons whose value generally continues throughout life.

Future projections

Early in the group, once there is at least a rudimentary sense of cohesion and as part of setting personal goals for the work, the leader(s) may direct members in a future projection exercise. Through a process as simple as having everyone stand and walk around their chairs in a clockwise direction, or as complicated as a guided visualization of the passage of time, members are led (in surplus reality) to "time travel" to the final meeting of the group. The leader(s) may then say something like, "Well, here we are at the final session of our group. Let's take a look at what we have accomplished and what we wish we could have done but did not." Group members can then voice their thoughts about these matters.

Using future projection rather than asking members, "What do you hope you will get from the group and what do you think you want to get but won't achieve?" has several advantages. In terms of laying a foundation for good termination, it reinforces from the start that this group is going to end. This exercise also allows members to try on their feelings about ending while there is still a good percentage of group time remaining. Additionally, participation in this activity helps create a vested interest in the outcome of each member's commitment to make the group all it can be.

The imagination is a powerful tool, and using theirs the members create a template of success first in surplus reality; later, they can use this as a guide to build actual reality in real time. Asking questions such as "What were some of the steps we made along the way that helped us get here?" can also provide an outline of an action plan for the group as each member begins articulating his or her personal goals and objectives.

While in the surplus reality of the last group meeting, members can also be asked "How do you generally handle endings?" After this and any other pertinent questions have been answered, members return in time (moving counter-clockwise around the chairs or through another visualization).

Once fully back in the present, members can be asked what they will need to do to create the outcomes they envisioned and also to have this group's ending be a different kind of experience than any unproductive ones they may have had.

Setting incremental goals

During the goals and objectives setting activities, members can be asked to set a series of successive and incremental goals to be evaluated along the way. With a group that lasts the entire school year, for example, members can be asked what they hope to accomplish by various breaking points in the school year, coinciding with various holidays or vacations. In this manner, goals can be articulated in a way that is realistic as well as measurable, while members can begin warming up to the idea that there will be a series of endings and beginnings that will lead up to the final ending.

Rehearsals for ending

Throughout the group's time together, a number of opportunities may arise to "practice" healthy termination behavior. The ability to have "clean" and productive endings is an important adult skill. Each issue or trial that is met by the group concerning endings helps this skill to develop.

Warming up to holidays

In the groups I conducted in New Hampshire, we always took extended breaks during certain public and school holidays. The approach of each of these vacation times provided an opportunity to practice termination skills.

SOCIODRAMA AND PSYCHODRAMA

Sociodramas and/or psychodramatic vignettes can be enacted about the kinds of stressors, general or specific, as well as fun events that are likely to occur during the time in which the group is not meeting. Members can practice various tactics for dealing with the stressors, including phoning each other for support. It is important to check out with each member what the acceptable parameters are for him or her about making and receiving phone calls so that this tactic does not add to family stress.

Although members know that they will be returning to group after a week or two, they have the opportunity to practice how they can take the support structures they have been developing with them even when the group is not meeting. Holiday times can be extremely difficult without support, and so this work serves a vital function in present time as well as in rehearsing for the actual ending of the group.

SANTA'S WORKSHOP

As the group moves toward the December holidays, if the tradition of Santa Claus is one appropriate to the membership, an activity based on the psychodramatic structure known as *Magic Shop* (Leveton 2001) can be used. In this version, members have the opportunity to visit *Santa's Workshop* to ask for any "nonphysical" gift they would like to receive for the holiday season; for example, peace in the family, more patience with younger siblings, etc. A series of sculptures or vignettes can be constructed, using "Santa's elves" (group members) as auxiliaries, to show both what it looks like when the family is in turmoil and what it would look like if the holiday were peaceful. Costumes can add to the festive nature of the activity if desired.

As with the Magic Shop, Santa's gift does not come for free; there must be an exchange. The shopper needs to discover what they have that they can leave at least a portion of with Santa in exchange for their gift. Perhaps it is a generous portion of "argumentative nature" or "older sibling arrogance." As they work on the exchange, they discover personal tactics that can help them achieve their goals.

Leave of absence

There may also be instances, with groups that run for longer periods of time, when members or group leaders need to take a leave of absence for any number of reasons.

A MEMBER'S LEAVE OF ABSENCE

A member's taking a leave of absence provides the member with practice in assembling ways to make the support of the group "portable" and for the remaining members to express their feelings about the departure productively.

In one group I conducted, a member was taking a leave in order to take drivers' education classes that were being given after school. The member could not afford private classes that were offered in the evening and really needed to have a driver's license to be able to get a job, since he lived outside of town and there was no public transportation available.

Unfortunately, he was also having a lot of difficulty at home and would miss the support the group was providing. Group members were upset that he would not be there for eight weeks, because they were really involved in doing some intense work and wanted him to be a part of it.

As group members expressed both their support as well as distress about his leaving, they offered a psychodramatic gift for him to take to support him in his family struggles, for example, patience, a sense of humor, and the knowledge that there were friends who cared. He made a nametag that could be placed on an empty chair to hold his place while he was gone. He also promised to send notes to the group each week that could be read at the start of group. Furthermore, he offered to see how many absences he was allowed over the eight weeks of three days a week of drivers' education classes and from that information he would see if he could take his "excused absences" on group meeting days so that he would not have to miss every group meeting for the entire eight weeks. For him as well as for the group, this process of negotiating and planning for his leave was probably as beneficial as it would have been for him to have had uninterrupted attendance.

A LEADER'S LEAVE OF ABSENCE

A leader taking a leave of absence can stir up a lot of feeling for group members. Even if there will only be one session missed, it is important to let the group know in advance. When the leader is going to be gone for a longer period of time, more indepth work needs to be done, not only to provide members with the opportunity to express feelings, but also to look at the roles that the leader holds in the group and at who will hold them during the absence.

In 2001, I took a three-month sabbatical from my group leader and administrative roles with ACTINGOUT. The groups began in early October and ran through mid-May. I was gone December through February. For the groups that contained new members, the process involved making sure that the co-leaders of the groups (graduate interns) played a strong co-leadership role from the first group meeting. This set up the situation that could be framed "one of our leaders is leaving." With the members who were in continuing groups, the situation was different. These members had worked with me for at least one previous program year and some for as many as eight consecutive years. In one of these groups, there was a co-leader who was a staff member with whom most members also had an ongoing relationship, but the graduate interns were in the role of "itinerant leaders." For these groups, the frame was "our primary, long-term leader is leaving."

The process we evolved was similar for all the groups, but adapted to take into account the strength of attachment members had to me as representing their ongoing connection to their participation in the program. I will describe here the process as it was used with the group composed of older members and those of longest standing.

Part of the process from the start of the group year, after announcing the sabbatical, was to provide lots of opportunities for expression of feelings. Some was done in group discussion, with people offering both expressions of fear about "what would happen without Mario's strong leadership" as well as encouragement for my trip to Australia and appreciation for my modeling of self-care. In sessions of nondirected improvisation (more a drama therapy than psychodrama approach), stronger feelings emerged and could be contained in the safety of the scenes. I played the "abandoning parent," and was scolded and yelled at for not caring. From within the role, I could offer validation of the feelings as well as the assurance that I would return and my faith that "my children" were "mature enough" to take care of themselves and one another for a time.

To address the specific concerns about how the group would function without "Mario's strong leadership," we decided to focus on the roles that I played as a leader and how these role functions would be shared in my absence. Sticky notes were given to the members and they wrote on them all the roles they could think of that I carried for them and the group: "good-enough father," "obsessive organizer," "caring challenger," etc. Each group member named aloud the roles they had written as they stuck them on the shirt I was wearing. The next step was for me to then name each role and ask who in the group, among the leaders and members, could take responsibility for that role function in my absence. Some roles required two people, some needed only one. Some of the roles, it was realized, were already possessed by others in their own way. With some of the roles, for example, the "wise grandfather," members realized that this particular role would be unfilled, for a time. The role assignments were recorded on a piece of poster board so they could be visibly present during group meetings.

I had also brought into the group a gnarled piece of driftwood that I had found. It was fairly thick and quite smooth. Each member wrote the roles they had named on the stick. This became the "Mario Stick," and would be available to be used as a talking object (a Native American tradition that supports one person's speaking at a time) or just to hold my place on an empty chair so the group could appreciate my presence even though I would be absent.

In addition, group members set goals for what they wanted to accomplish while I was gone. Thanks to the "magic" of e-mail, I was able to send regular messages to the groups during my absence. I also provided supervision to the leaders to support their process with the groups.

I am happy to report that all survived, even thrived, in my absence. Upon my return, I was welcomed back through a process of reclaiming roles. With some roles, it was noticed that others had developed them sufficiently and that I didn't need to take them back, or at least not to the same degree that I had held them before.

Unexpected departures

There are also times in the life of a group during which members or leaders leave unexpectedly. In some cases, they share the reason with the group and attend at least a final session before departing. In other cases, they just stop coming, without communicating their intention to the group in some way. Supporting the group to have appropriate closure with these departing members is another piece of developing clear termination skills.

In the event that the group is notified in advance and the departing member or leader comes to a final session, it is important to allow group members to express their full range of feelings about the departure. If the feelings include anger and/or disappointment, the leader(s) needs to be thoughtful about supporting expression of the feelings without blaming the person departing or having the session focus on trying to get the person to change his or her mind. Using "I" statements and other good communication skills can be important. Supporting the departing member or leader in expressing their feelings fully is also important. In cases in which the decision to leave is beyond their control, the departing member may have a great deal of grief, frustration or anger to express themselves. Of course, if the person departing is a leader, their focus should be more on how their sharing of feelings supports the group and save their own needs for a time of closure with other staff.

Departing members can be offered a future projection psychodramatic vignette in which they practice drawing on skills they have developed during their time in the group to help them in some potentially stressful life situations in their future. Or group members can create a group sculpture of what the group will become when this member is gone.

Even if the group is one focused on a specific task or issue, termination becomes the task or issue of the group during these times. To short-change the termination process because there is "work to be done" misses the real value of the group experience as a microcosm of life experience.

In the event that a member leaves without coming to say goodbye, or in some cases without even notifying the group of the intended departure, the group still must deal with the issue of termination. During my early years as a group therapist, there was a member who had been in a car accident and was doing all right in recovery for a few days, and then unexpectedly died. Although this is an extreme example, there is a need for closure with those who leave unexpectedly in any manner. After the death of that member, as well as at times of other unfinished departures, an empty chair was used to represent the person so that the group members could express their goodbyes. In the case of the member who had died, there was the chance to express all the things "I wish I had said to you," as well as the sorrow and grief and even anger that were felt. With other departures, especially if some of the group members would still have contact with the departed member, it was important to keep the focus on the remaining members expressing their feelings and not have it become a put-down session in absentia.

Terminating the group

Truly, issues of termination begin at the first group session, and the wise and thoughtful leader recognizes opportunities along the way to support the process of termination rather than waiting until the last few sessions to deal with it.

As groups approach their final sessions, provided that appropriate work has been done all along, the members are more likely to engage in active work around termination issues. Members can be warmed up with an Opening Circle question, such as: "How do you normally deal with endings?" Once stated, members can explore their typical responses to endings and then see if they want to try something different. If this question was originally asked during a future projection activity at the beginning of the group, it may still be used in real time, as the answers may well have changed. It may be interesting, if any notes or records of that future projection session exist, to compare the answers during or after this "real-time" session.

Timeline activities

It is important for group members to reflect on where they have come, individually and as a group, from their first to final sessions. A timeline can be set up in the action space and individuals or the entire group can move along it and reflect on the issues and struggles and victories they have encountered along the way. A line can be made on the floor with masking tape, using hash marks at various intervals to mark significant events. At other times, particularly if individuals are reviewing their progress, colored scarves can be employed to represent the various challenges encountered even though not necessarily in strict chronological order. Timelines can be explored as a series of dialogues, monologues or soliloquies. Or this activity may be accomplished nonverbally, with members or the group creating a series of sculptures depicting the various points along the way.

As the group and its members recall the victories they have had along with the challenges, they can draw encouragement for continuing to be successful with the current challenge of ending well. The timeline can also be projected into the future, with places assigned for a week after the group is over, for a month, etc. Members can project how they will carry the work they have done into their day-to-day lives, or for important upcoming occasions, such as graduation, moving, starting a job, beginning or changing colleges, weddings, and so on.

Giving feedback

Activities that allow members to reflect on how well they have done in achieving their goals and to receive feedback from the leader(s) and other group members are also appropriate at this juncture. One possible structure is the use of the *hot seat*. A chair is placed in the action space and, as they are ready, members sit in it for self-reflection and feedback. Members first reflect on how well they feel they have done in achieving their goals, what unexpected challenges they have dealt with and with what degree of success. They then ask the group for feedback, if they want it, and let the group know what kind of feedback they want as well as how "honest" or "direct" they want the feedback to be. A member can ask for positive feedback only, and their request is honored. Few will do this, but having the degree of candor to be in each recipient's control allows for the celebration of his or her ability to hear constructive feedback, as well as for the feedback itself.

Leaders can participate in offering feedback as well as in receiving it from the group. It is generally a sound policy for leaders to offer their feedback last, so that members have a full opportunity to express their feelings, and so the leader can pick up those points that might have been missed that would be clinically appropriate for the member to hear, both positive and constructive.

Reclaiming roles

During participation in groups, members and leaders hold many different roles for each other. The leader may be cast in the role of the "good-enough parent" or the "caring aunt or uncle." Other members may be the "loving sibling" or the "friend and confidante." These roles have been projected and accepted perhaps because the members don't have them in their lives, need more of them, or need to find them outside of their current support system. Whatever the case, members need an opportunity to reclaim roles that they must now hold for themselves, or make a "shopping list" for the kinds of healthy relationships they will seek outside of the group. It may be that relationships with other group members will continue. If so, members should be encouraged to continue these relationships consciously and think about the differences between being a "loving sibling" or "friend and confidante" outside of the group and within it.

An activity similar to the one I described earlier that was used when I went on sabbatical is one possibility for working with these role transitions. It would make the roles more clear and help members evaluate which they are ready to take on for themselves, which still require another person to hold, and which may be no longer needed.

In 2003, when I left ACTINGOUT and brought to a close the relationships with a number of participants that had been sustained over a number of years, the process of role reclamation was extremely important. The process took place over the course of the entire program year (from September through May). Early in the program year, when the group members were each creating a sculpture of the group as they saw it, one member had placed me with my back to the group and heading out the door. This was a vivid reminder that issues around my leaving would be a part of the ongoing process of the group for the entire year.

As the year came to an end, a weekend "retreat" was held with these members, and each had several hours in which to do the psychodrama of their choice. Many brought me into the drama to participate in a ritual of claiming back the roles I had held for them over the years. Ironically, I was suffering from a severe case of laryngitis at the time and had been ordered to observe complete vocal rest (no talking at all). My interaction was limited to gesture and what could be written down. In many ways, my silence helped keep the focus on the members. One role that I had held for many of them over the years was the "thoughtful articulator," one who could find the words to express what was happening in the moment. In these dramas, members reclaimed that role. A symbolic display of this role transition came at a farewell performance given in my honor a short time later. These same group members served as my "voice" to express the feelings and ideas that I wanted to share with the community.

The importance of grieving

While it is vital to support members in claiming roles and abilities they take with them from the group, and celebrating the victories and struggles they have had along the way, it is also vital to grieve. Endings are a part of life and do mark new beginnings, and they are often sad. We support our group members in claiming their fully functioning adult roles by supporting the expression of a full range of feelings.

Some might debate the appropriateness of leaders crying right along with group members at the endings of groups. In my opinion, if the tears are genuine and not forced, I believe they are appropriate and healthy, as long as the leaders' crying does not "upstage" the members' tears. Over the years, I have shared many a box of tissues with group members, but never to the point that the members felt they had to "take care of" me. With those boundaries in place, members may feel freer to share their grief, as they can see that adults as well as adolescents experience feelings of loss expressed in tears.

This reality is also crucial to model: grief is intense, uncomfortable, and often painful, but it is not dangerous, unlimited, bottomless, or a cause for terror. In fact, as has been shown by many researchers and by our own personal experiences, pure grief, untainted by these other more problematic responses, is actually cleansing, somewhat soothing, and natural. When group members and leaders share, within clear boundaries, whatever naturally arises for them regarding any types of terminations or losses in such a group, this paves the way for all members to handle future grieving in healthy ways.

Summary

At each stage of group development, members face challenges as well as opportunities to enhance or expand upon their adult life skills. The process of termination begins with the first group, and foundations for healthy termination can be laid during future projection and *goal-setting activities*. Throughout the life of the group, there are opportunities to practice healthy endings in action, as members warm up for and deal with holidays as well as leaves of absence and departures of members and/or leaders.

As the group comes to a close, it is important for members to grieve fully as well as to review their accomplishments and struggles, receive feedback, and reclaim and re-evaluate roles. At each step of the way, action techniques offer the adolescent group an enriching experience.

There are several important subjects yet to be covered, such as how to incorporate action techniques with specific kinds of populations, and how to apply the ideas from this book in varied and actual settings by group leaders from diverse backgrounds and traditions. These are explored in Part III.

Part III

Sharing: Other Applications of Action Techniques and Considerations for their Implementation

Part I of this book explored both the philosophical and theoretical underpinnings of action techniques in general as well as their utilization with adolescent groups. It reviewed individual and group developmental stages and their relationships to each other as well as some of the specific developmental challenges of adolescence. Part I also explored the importance of good leadership and clear group norms for creating a "safe space" within which a group can work.

Part II presented suggestions for using action techniques to meet the special challenges of each stage of group development as well as action techniques and information that speak to the developmental challenges of adolescence that can be addressed during each stage. The appendices supplement this information.

Part III explores ways in which the material from Parts I and II can be applied with "special populations" and in diverse settings. It also contains insights about the importance for group leaders of integrating their own theoretical and philosophical beliefs with their practice of action techniques. Additionally, it offers items for group leaders to consider in responding to the fluctuating nature of adolescent group member behavior and practical considerations for developing and implementing action groups for adolescence.

CHAPTER 9

Adapting Action Techniques to the Population and Setting

Action techniques are applicable to adolescent groups throughout their stages of development. In the best of all possible worlds, counselors and therapists who work with young people would be able to design and implement their group meeting plans to take full advantage of the power of action and its suitability to their participants. Unfortunately, realities of agency budgets and policies and managed care, as well as the vagaries of politics, often mean settling for less than the ideal. Compromises must be made, and alterations to "ideal" plans must occur.

Just as it is vital to understand the ways in which adolescents are different from adults, so is it vital to understand that certain groups of adolescents may present special challenges or considerations in using action techniques. So too do certain settings. The core philosophy and theory remain the same, but modifications may be necessary in the implementation of certain techniques. Cultural and/or regional considerations may require adapting an approach that worked well in one part of the world or with one cultural group in order to serve better in another location. This chapter explores some of these considerations.

I present first considerations about particular types of youth populations. Next, I explore various settings. This chapter is intended not so much to be a training manual for working with these populations nor for working in these settings, but rather to serve as a review of things to keep in mind when using action techniques under these circumstances. I also include ideas for the uses of specific kinds of action strategies with specific populations. Because I have selected populations and settings on the basis of my knowledge of and experience with them, this selection is by no means inclusive of all possibilities. The major focus remains, as it does throughout the book, on therapeutic applications in clinical settings.

Working with special populations

When young people are separated into subgroups within an institution or agency because of shared characteristics, these subgroupings are what I am calling "special populations." In some therapeutic or educational environments, adolescents are grouped or segregated on the basis of certain distinguishing characteristics, such as learning needs, behavioral problems, or mental health diagnoses. In other situations, young people with "special needs" are "mainstreamed" into programs within the general population. Recognizing that there are advantages as well as disadvantages to working with either homogeneous or heterogeneous groupings of young people, whatever the balance or composition of the group, leaders should approach each group with awareness of the needs of all the members, however diverse. The following sections, though not exhaustive in scope, cover a variety of special populations and the considerations that should be taken into account when incorporating action techniques while designing and implementing programs for these young people.

Young people with attention deficit disorder (ADD) and attention deficit / hyperactivity disorder (ADHD)

When I first heard the term "attention deficit disorder," my immediate reaction was, "Isn't that interesting? There are diagnostic criteria for kids who are disordered because they did not get enough attention." Very soon I realized my error, but the original misapprehension struck me as significant. After working for many years in groups with members who carried the label ADD or ADHD, I have come to realize that the problems these young people encounter have more to do with reciprocity of attention than is recognized by the diagnostic criteria for this disorder in its "official" definition.

I have worked with groups of adolescents in which a number of members carried this diagnosis. Many of them were taking medication during the school day to try to make their behavior more "manageable" for teachers. Provided that these young people genuinely wanted to be a part of the group, we were almost always able to work out strategies that allowed these members to participate fully without their having to take another dosage of their medication after school, despite recommended dosages.

One reason I believe our strategies were so successful with these types of young people is that action approaches are ideal for this population because they do not require group members to "sit still" for long periods of time. The group is up and moving frequently, and the action changes as the group session progresses.

Another advantageous strategy is that group norms can be structured so that, even during times in which members are sitting and talking, a member who needs to is allowed to get up and move around, as long as it is done in a way that minimizes disruption. All group members can practice various techniques for "nondisruptive roving" without ever having to disclose who carries which diagnosis. Any member may feel and then fulfill a need to move about from time to time.

Furthermore, "going with a member's strength" may mean that group members are encouraged to find things to do with their hands that fulfill a need for fidgeting without making disruptive noise. Playing with clay, doodling, or squeezing a soft rubber ball may serve this purpose nicely. Interesting artwork often emerges from these proceedings which later may become relevant to the group's activities. Members can be enlisted in exploring their particular needs and discovering novel and workable solutions that will maximize their chances for successful group participation.

Learning to contain (see Part II for extensive descriptions of containment) is also important for these young people, and clear norms and boundaries must be stated and enforced. A leader may need to sit near certain members to coach or support them in prearranged ways so they can have a greater chance of success. With extreme cases, I have even used *out of control tokens*. Members are told that if they stray too far from the norms or become disruptive, they will be given a token and asked to calm down. Three tokens acquired in one session warrant a *time out*. Although it might seem odd to employ a "behavioral" approach in an expressive therapy group, my experience is that it has worked. Within a few sessions, the members in need of this technique learned how to manage their behavior to remain within acceptable norms. ADD or ADHD teens who were able to remain members of an expressive arts group for several consecutive years benefited greatly from this experience.

I remember one instance, during a field trip, when I was walking next to one of my older, long-term group members, one who had initially been a prototypic ADHD adolescent. He looked at a newer member of the group who was behaving in an extremely hyperactive manner, then said to me, "Hey, remember when I used to be like that?"

The condition itself can be the subject for a drama, in which the group member gets to confront ADD as a concretized character, dialog with it, and work out a new contract or job description that gradually shifts control from the disorder to the member. The ADD/ADHD members can explore "triggers" that tend to precede periods of disordered thinking and behavior and work on strategies for dealing with these problems in "socially acceptable" ways.

I fear that much of what has originally been diagnosed as ADD or ADHD in school settings is more accurately labeled a "reasonable reaction to a nonengaging classroom." Some schools simply do not employ sufficiently diverse or effective pedagogies and so do not acknowledge and/or address the various learning styles and preferences of their students. Then, rather than recognizing that the responsibility for managing these needs resides with the institution and its "expert" staff, the staff blame the students for being unable to learn. Alternatively, when we observe or work with young people who are engaged fully in what they are doing, for example, who are working on learning a new skateboard maneuver, doing artwork, listening to their favorite music, or participating in dramatic action, it is difficult to tell which of them carries the ADD brand. So, it is not that these students cannot; it is that, given the right circumstances, they may participate fully and attentively.

Suicidal young people

It is not unusual for adolescents to have suicidal thoughts. Fortunately, not all thoughts lead to action. It is important for adolescents to know that they are not alone in thinking "dark" thoughts. Suicide or suicidal thoughts should be discussed openly when they arise in groups. Any counselor or therapist working with young people (or any other population, for that matter) should have training and supervision around the appropriate and safe ways to support clients who are suicidal.

It is also important to know that there are laws that leaders are required to follow concerning mandated reporting of group members' intentions to harm self or others. Leaders must make all reporting requirements known to group members during the beginning meetings, and differentiate these topics clearly from other information that can remain confidential within the group. Then, when a reportable incident occurs, leaders should discuss the incident and its reporting with the member individually and the group as a whole.

It is not my intention here to train the reader in accepted suicide intervention strategies. Rather, I will present some action strategies for addressing this issue if and when it does arise in the course of a group session.

GROUP MEMBERS' REACTIONS TO SUICIDE

Suicide often becomes an issue for the group when a family member or acquaintance of some members commits suicide. Suicidal thinking also often arises in the aftermath of peer death due to accidents or other tragedies, or as a reaction to some teens' extreme difficulties in their own lives. Suicide definitely becomes a group issue when any group members share that they have been thinking about killing themselves.

In the case of the suicide of a friend or family member, it is important to provide a venue for the expression of feelings that are stirred for the survivors. The suicide of one young person will often raise suicidal thoughts in others, whether or not they were part of the departed person's social circle. As these thoughts arise, they should be dealt with openly and honestly.

Certainly a safety assessment should be conducted if any member is at risk of acting on these thoughts. However, contrary to popular fears and misconceptions, talking about suicide does not make suicidal action more likely, as long as these conversations are conducted in a thoughtful manner.

A group may utilize either psychodramatic or sociodramatic methods in working with reactions to suicide; this decision often depends both upon the stage of group development that the group is currently in and the experience levels of members with action methods. Here are some action methods for managing the topic of suicide in a group setting.

Working psychodramatically

As discussed previously, an empty chair can be used to represent an absent or dead individual, such as the suddenly departed person. Psychodramatic techniques which allow rotating protagonists would allow each volunteering member to address his or her feelings to the "person" in the chair. It is wise to let members know overtly that it is all right to express feelings of anger and outrage, since these feelings will generally be present but internally perceived prohibitions against such expression may keep a member stuck, or unwilling to express these feelings without support.

I generally do *not* engage members in role reversal with the deceased. I believe that this is more likely to lead to feelings of guilt or to spark suicidal thoughts for the member, rather than provide a cathartic experience. I might have a leader or noninvolved group member take on the role to assure the survivor that it was not his/her fault.

Working sociodramatically

In cases where the members' connection to a recent suicide is peripheral, but the topic still needs to be addressed, a sociodramatic approach can be employed. The characters might be "a suicidal teen" and "a caring friend." The group can work together to generate a list of life situations that may lead someone to considering suicide. As members take on the "suicidal teen" role, they can be assigned a situation that *does not* correspond to a current life issue for them. As members take on the "caring friend" role, they can practice and evaluate various strategies for supporting a friend who is in this type of crisis. It is important for the leader to stress both how important the support of a friend can be in this situation, as well as the fact that adult support should be sought if one has a suicidal friend, regardless of whether or not the friend has asked that nothing be said to anyone. As with the exceptions to confidentiality in the group, even with friends, there are some secrets that should not be kept.

It is also worth mentioning that, no matter now well-intentioned, no person can truly prevent another from harming themselves if that person is determined to do so. It is important to state clearly that the "suicidal teen's" death, if it occurs from suicide, is *not* the "caring friend's" fault.

SUICIDAL MEMBER(S) WITHIN THE GROUP

In the case of a group member's disclosure of suicidal thoughts, although the problem now resides "within" the group, and "within" an individual, the approach may still be either sociodramatic or psychodramatic.

A sociodramatic approach

An intrapsychic sociodrama can be set up to support the suicidal group member. For this drama, the roles are: "a group member"; "the part of self that holds strongly to life"; and "the part that thinks about dying." The leader should be sure that each member who participates takes a turn in the "self" chair, with a statement of where they are in the moment. By approaching the issue sociodramatically, even if there is only one member who is feeling suicidal, leaders allow for unspoken thoughts to be revealed and also give the suicidal member the opportunity to view the issues from an observing perspective, providing additional training for the Observing Ego role.

During the drama, the leader(s) can be conducting a preliminary safety assessment for members who are in the "thinking-about-dying" role as well as the "life" role, to determine whether to do contracting for no self-harm or reporting for each member.

A psychodramatic approach

The following is an example of a psychodramatic intervention used in a fairly experienced group with a suicidal member. The group member, let's call her Wanda, had asked for some "group time" during check-in. She shared with the group that the previous evening she had been feeling so low that she was seriously considering suicide. There were a number of factors: boyfriend, school, and family stress among them. She reported sitting there with a bottle of sleeping pills in her hand and a glass of water at her side. She told the group that the only reason she didn't take the pills was that she didn't want to upset the group.

I had a brief discussion with Wanda, the group, and my co-leader. We then set up the following drama. The group sat in a circle with my co-leader. Wanda and I sat on the stage, outside of the group. The drama began with my co-leader telling the group that Wanda had committed suicide. Wanda and I sat in "the spirit world" and watched each member's reaction. The group was very focused on the drama, with none of the giggles or silliness that could have occurred. The expression of feelings was intense. At times, Wanda tried to say something to a particular member, but of course they could not hear her.

By the time the drama was finished, there wasn't (as the saying goes) a "dry eye in the house." The sharing that followed was very rich and offered the members a chance to talk about their own dark feelings as well as their genuine desire to support Wanda. Wanda was amazed at the degree of caring that was available to her from the group. She also had the opportunity, in surplus reality, to reflect on the wisdom of her choice after the fact. She agreed to a "no self-harm" contract as well as a plan to check in with a different member of the group by phone each evening.

This session was a turning point for Wanda and her work in the group. She remained a committed member throughout high school and often told new members about how the group had "saved her life."

Suicidal thoughts are common for young people, and their expression must be taken seriously, even though the leader realizes that not all thoughts will lead to action. Local organizations that deal with youth suicide can provide resources for the leader and will often provide speakers to work with groups, thoughtfully and appropriately, on this issue.

Just as working with suicide and suicidal youth is something that group leaders need special training in, working with young people (or adults) who lack a well-formed conscience, or who have exhibited sociopathic characteristics, also demands intensive, specialized training. In the next section, far from providing this extensive training, I do offer some insights and activities that may prove helpful for leaders that have groups that include such young people.

Antisocial and sociopathic young people

As mentioned previously, there are some prerequisites – conditions that must be present for each member – in order to work effectively in a group setting. At a minimum, youth participants must be able both to give and receive attention (be able to listen and to respond) and to possess some basic social skills, such as being willing to agree and adhere to group norms. Lacking these fundamental abilities, many young people who are considered "antisocial" or "sociopathic" are not good candidates for large group work. Many of them lack even the most rudimentary sense of empathy, hence are unable to feel or show remorse for their actions. Additionally, the expansive nature of many action techniques may be counterproductive with individuals who need to learn containment.

Action techniques, however, can be employed in working individually or in very small groups with these young people to focus on role training for prosocial behavior. Through role reversal, they may begin to develop a sense of empathy. Through role play, they may broaden their repertoire of possible responses and begin to develop missing skills of appropriate social interaction. If in a group setting, working sociodramatically rather than psychodramatically will be the preferred mode, until many intrapsychic strengths and greatly improved empathic abilities are in place for all members.

For the leaders, knowledge and experience in working with this population, as well as skill and experience in the methodology, are essential. Robson (2000), in writing about her work using psychodrama with adolescent sexual offenders, offers some good insights for those who work with this type of population.

It is also important to enforce group norms consistently and strongly for the benefit and safety of the other group members. When an antisocial member is drawing a lot of attention during a group meeting, the leader can become so focused on trying to help that one member have a successful experience that the contract with other members is violated. There are times that it is more appropriate to remove a member from the group and then make arrangements for individual work for the good of both that member and the group. It is about finding the appropriate venue for someone's work, not blaming the member being removed or framing it as a "failure."

Young victims of childhood trauma

As mentioned at the end of Chapter 7, it is difficult and probably ill-advised to work in action on specific issues of childhood trauma with any types of adolescent clients. The most important thing to consider in working with young people in this category is to focus on identifying and strengthening the healthy roles and abilities that the trauma has prevented them from developing fully throughout their history. As detailed in Part II, action techniques can be well employed to work with young people on any of the unmet developmental challenges of childhood as well as to approach the challenges of adolescence. The group experience, however, can be an extremely therapeutic one for these young people. Action techniques can support them in reclaiming their power and their ability to connect to their own and one another's strengths.

I worked with a young woman who had been a victim of incest. Her manner was generally withdrawn and her voice unusually soft. During a sociodrama on the issue of abusive relationships, she "found her voice" and claimed her right to be treated with respect. This was a turning point in her treatment, her recovery, and healing, even though we were not directly dealing with her life issues.

Even though some methods can be successful, working directly with trauma memories, even with adults, requires special training and experience. Once group members move into action, many of their usual defense mechanisms that provide them some protection during more traditional "talk" therapy may be outmaneuvered. This makes members extremely vulnerable, and therefore also at risk of encountering a variety of adverse consequences during and from this experience.

Additionally, by putting any elements (setting, roles, events, related memories) of a personal trauma into action, the risk for retraumatization is great. In a group comprised of many survivors or those involved in current experiences of abuse or trauma, playing any role in or even watching such a drama can retraumatize those members.

The reader interested in this area of work is referred to Kellermann and Hudgins (2000) and Hudgins (2002) for more indepth reviews of utilizing psychodrama with survivors of trauma.

Differently abled young people

There are advantages in having "differently abled" youth as participants in a group of "regularly abled" youth. The advantages extend to all the group members, regardless of their abilities or disabilities. The only real requirements for group participation were listed earlier: a potential member must be able to give and receive attention, and she or he must have rudimentary social skills.

I have worked in groups with members who were "legally" blind, were somewhat developmentally delayed, and had speech impediments. These members were incredibly committed to their groups and gained tremendously from being in a setting in which they could be "part of the crowd." It did take time, and other group members were sometimes slow to warm up to the idea, or were overprotective and patronizing. Everyone, however, benefited from including these members.

With support from the leaders and occasional coaching, the "differently abled" members were able to be present in role for their fellow group members with a sincerity and clarity of focus that were commendable for any adolescent. There was no observable limitation for any of these members in their ability to participate in group activities, once appropriate accommodations were made. It is important for leaders to assist all group members to distinguish which accommodations are required and then to make them versus knowing which responses are patronizing or limiting towards the disabled members and to refrain from making those.

Furthermore, as the "differently abled" members shared their stories about what it was like to be the "blind girl" or to be teased for being different, other members began to make the connection between these stories and their own. Each member had experienced being picked on or feeling different at one time or another. The specifics became less important than the core issues. Being the "goth" in a "preppy" class did not feel so different from being the "blind girl" in a "sighted" class. In time, not only were the "differently abled" members treated like everybody else (for good and ill), but the distinctions all but disappeared and all became "peers," sometimes for the first times in their lives.

Substance abusing young people

Action strategies are extremely effective and important for working with young people on issues of substance abuse. They can be used to explore the ownership of the problem and degree of abuse as well as in rehearsals for sober behavior.

EXPLORING THE PROBLEM

An effective strategy for exploring a young person's relationship to a substance is to set aside the value judgment and focus on the relationship. One way to become clear about the nature of abuse is to explore the ways in which the relationship to the substance gets in the way of relationships to people and other things in the young person's life. A psychodramatic vignette can be set up in which the substance using group member creates a scene with his or her substance, personified into the role of "Mary Wanna," "Jack Daniels," or "Nick O'Tien." The focus of the scene could be on the protagonist's "breaking off" the relationship. Through role reversal with the substance, the participant can gain a better understanding of the hold this substance has over him or her, analogous to the dynamics of an abusive relationship.

If working with a number of substance using/abusing young people at once, each can take the role of their substance of choice and appear as guests on a talk show; the rest of the group plays the audience members. With good facilitation, a psycho-sociodrama of this sort can be a lot of fun and provide a good deal of insight. Once the substance playing group members are solidly in their roles, the "host" of the talk show can inform them that, before coming on the program, they were each given a delayed action truth serum in their coffee and so all questions from that moment forward must be answered truthfully. Casting the "audience members" as "recovering addicts" and encouraging them to question and challenge the "guests" adds dimension and energy to the drama, as well as providing maximum involvement of the entire group.

It is important with this type of activity to de-role each member fully and allow them to return to the role of self when the drama has ended (see Appendix D for de-roling activities). They also ought to have a chance to make a final statement to the substance concerning the future of the relationship. Not every group member will be ready to end the relationship, but perhaps their negotiating for a different relationship can be their next step in dealing with the problem.

SUPPORTING RECOVERY THROUGH ROLE TRAINING

Substance abusing young people have lots of practice with the role of the "user" or "addict." Even when highly motivated to work at recovery, they need practice with roles that promote sobriety. I have done psychodramatic work at inpatient, substance abuse treatment programs for adolescents. A vital part of the process, especially for those patients who were soon to be released, was to practice behaviors that supported recovery.

In creating scenes of this nature, it is much better to use staff or team members to play the needed "user friend" or "tempter" roles so as to diminish the hold these roles already have over the young person. Often, while negotiating a scene about declining a substance when visiting old friends, the person in recovery will realize that they must stay away from friends who are still using, and so the role training becomes about declining the invitation over the phone or from the friend one meets at the mall.

Sobriety Shop (Rustin and Olsson 1993), a variation on the Magic Shop technique referenced in Chapter 8, provides an opportunity "in which personal qualities that have contributed to the patient's addictive illness are exchanged for desirable qualities that will help the patient stay sober" (p.12). For example, dishonesty can be traded for honesty, or insecurity for self-esteem. Unlike the caveat in traditional Magic Shop, the item traded in does not have to be one of value that other shoppers would want, just one that does not serve the participant's recovery. However, like dishonesty, the quality might have been of great service to maintaining the role of the addict.

Young people with eating disorders

Creating opportunities for young people with eating disorders to communicate with their disorder (anorexia or bulimia) can be extremely enlightening. The same caveats apply here, however, regarding working first with vulnerable group members to develop strengths and beginning sociodramatically with less experienced participants. Once members are ready to work psychodramatically, I have found that some activities work extremely well. Here are some examples of psychodramatic work I have done with teens with eating disorders.

Through role reversal with the disorder, the young person can begin to understand the role the disorder plays in their life and the functions it serves. As this becomes clearer, the group member can begin to explore other ways to have these functions addressed. It is important to remove judgment from the encounter. Indeed, the disorder is generally an ally, albeit one whose tactics are damaging. The disorder may be the only ally the anorexic and bulimic group members have (or believe they have).

In working with extreme cases of anorexia, the participant may not have sufficient energy to remain standing for long periods of time, let alone to participate in action in the traditional way. During a workshop conducted with staff and inpatients in an adolescent unit of a psychiatric hospital, I addressed that situation by having the patient's psychiatrist act as her double. The scene was about the various and overwhelming responsibilities that this girl had taken on in her life: at home, in school, and in the community. As she described each one, group members took a large cushion and gave it to her double to carry. In a short period of time, the psychiatrist looked like the "camel" whose next cushion would be the "straw that would break its back."

With tears in her eyes, the young woman said, "She can't carry that load by herself. She needs help." The director asked, "Who can help her?" After the protagonist decided which responsibilities she was ready to let go of and which she needed to carry herself, she named various possible helpers, and other patients and staff members assumed the named helper roles and took some of the cushions.

When I returned to work with this group some months later, this young woman had gained weight, was no longer on a monitored eating program, and was nearing her discharge date. The action approach had helped her to discover what her core issues were and had provided her with motivation to seek support while maintaining control of her life situation. Additionally, the experience of serving as his patient's double provided the psychiatrist with a perspective into this young woman that helped him adjust his focus of treatment from trying to manage her behavior to developing a more therapeutic relationship.

Young people from differing cultures

Bringing together young people from differing cultures provides a rich experience for all concerned. Action methods can work wonderfully to provide communication that is not dependent on language. In many cases there is likely to be a mixture of "dominant" and "nondominant" cultures in such a group mix. This will call for thoughtfulness on several levels.

RESPECTING CULTURAL NORMS

As the group is developing and articulating norms, care must be taken to ascertain whether there are cultural norms that may not be obvious to members of the dominant culture that would make it difficult for members of the incoming group to participate in action in the same way as the local group. Norms around eye contact, touching, distance of personal space, stepping forward into the center of attention, and prescriptions about interaction with elders may all be relevant factors. Additionally, it may not be possible or appropriate for the members of the incoming culture to articulate these differences in norms. A bit of homework on the part of the leader is required so these details can be handled with sensitivity.

I remember one group experience I had in Australia in which it appeared to me that no one was interested in stepping into the protagonist position. In reality, there was an Asian group member who was quite warmed up and was standing as close to the center of the group as her custom would allow. For her, she was making quite a stretch, putting herself out that far. To my western eyes, no one was warmed up to action. Fortunately I had a co-leader who was aware of the cultural norms and was able to help me understand what was happening and to respond accordingly.

AWARENESS OF THE DRIVE TO "WESTERNIZE"

Around much of the planet, the western culture is the dominant culture. Hollywood movies can be seen just about anywhere on the globe, as can television programs from the USA or the UK. Western music is also widely heard. In many countries, when immigrants arrive, particularly those who are refugees, the push is to incorporate them into the dominant culture and teach them "how to act like us." It is also likely true for many immigrants, and possibly for refugees, that the western culture is seen as desirable. If the "parent" generation is not attracted to the western norm, their children may be or may choose to be in order to fit in with schoolmates.

While there is value in a group to help "newcomers" learn their way around, much of the personal and cultural strengths that have supported these individuals in their transition can too easily be lost. The thoughtful group leader can support the group's recognizing the rich opportunity present when new members from different cultures become part of the group. New members can be supported in learning new skills that will serve them in a new culture while being given the opportunity to recognize, appreciate and share their cultural heritages with the group.

While working in South Africa, I was intrigued and somewhat amazed to learn that this relatively new democracy has 11 "official" languages. At first, I wondered why this choice had been made; surely it made everything more complicated. During a psychodrama I directed in which the protagonist, a young man who spoke 9 of the 11 languages, was exploring his rage toward those who during the days of apartheid had tried to eliminate the tribal languages, it became clear to me. Each language represented a unique culture. To eliminate a language was to dismiss that culture and the richness it has to offer this emerging nation. As a westerner, I realized I had a great deal to learn about democracy.

RESPECTING RELIGIOUS OBSERVANCE ISSUES

It is also possible that some or all members of a group may be from a particular religious group or denomination with which the leader is not familiar. Issues of religious holidays, customs and observances need to be considered in planning and implementing the group. A conversation with a religious leader in the community can provide the background information needed to conduct the group with awareness.

If the group is being offered exclusively for members of a certain denomination, the leader, especially if not a member of that group, must be clear about the expectations of the sponsor. There may be issues around gender roles, for example, with which the leader does not agree. There may be topics that the sponsor does not wish to have group members challenge or explore independently. A clear contract agreed upon by the leader, sponsor, and the members is essential.

If the group is one with a mixed and varied religious/spiritual background, and in which transpersonal exploration by members is encouraged and supported, this should also be made clear in the information provided to parents before the start of the group.

As cultural matters are addressed with sensitivity, action approaches can provide a rich array of possibilities for those from the various cultures to exchange ideas and information about their heritage. Working through metaphor, with folk or fairy tales, for example, provides an opportunity to share tales from all participating cultures and notice similarities as well as differences. Culturally diverse groups provide young people with a rich environment within which developmental needs can be addressed while developing a less parochial view of the world than is often the case in groups with a homogeneous composition.

Other non-mainstream young people

Many young people do not fit into local cultural norms. This is generally the case for gay, lesbian, bisexual, transgendered, transsexual, and "questioning" adolescents (those still determining either their sexual orientation or gender identities or both), but it is also the case for whatever the local "minority" may be, whether based on race, style of dress, or religious persuasion. Action methods can serve an important function in helping these young people voice their fears and frustrations, as well as claiming their individuality and personal esteem.

I believe that it is better to work with a range of young people together rather than separating adolescents by "type" and thereby further isolating them. As was discussed with "differently abled" youth and young people from differing cultures, working in a heterogeneous setting allows old barriers to be crossed and offers "non-mainstream" young people chances to experience a sense of connection to their more mainstream peers. It is a broadening experience for all. I can recall a number of instances in which young people were able to move away from their homophobic backgrounds because of having participated in group meetings in which fellow group members with whom they had developed a close and trusting relationship came out as gay or bisexual.

One sociodramatic approach that can help all members of groups begin to understand the "other" more fully is to create a scene in surplus reality in which a "non-mainstream" situation is prevalent, is the norm: for example, a community in which 90 percent of the people are of a particular background. This kind of social role reversal allows the focus on the issue of inclusion/isolation to become the dominant driving force of the scene rather than on the local or current cultural norms about what is accepted or not.

During adolescence, the need to belong and feel connected is generally a major motivating force. For those young people who do not "fit in," feelings of isolation can be debilitating for the individual, and lead to behaviors that are "high risk" for both the individual and their communities. Groups that allow for expression and inclusion of all points of view are empowering, illuminating, and perhaps lifesaving.

Young people with theatre experience

Having young people with experience in theatre arts in an action group can offer both advantages and disadvantages. One might expect theatre-trained group members to have fewer inhibitions about entering into action and have more spontaneity to bring to the group. These expectations may well be true and can be used to good advantage by pairing the more experienced with the less experienced to offer support and encouragement for action exploration.

It is also possible that theatre-trained members, unless they have had genuine theatre training (as opposed to having been in a lot of plays), may try to "emote" or "pretend" feelings rather than work to get in touch with genuine feelings. They also may be so warmed up to action that they leave little room for others to participate.

In a group in which there is a wide range of theatre experience, it can be helpful to create a spectrogram of experience early in the group's development. Once members have arranged themselves along the continuum from "no experience" to "lots of experience," leaders could then interview the members at the extremes about what it feels like to be where they are and what their hopes and fears may be about those at the opposite extreme. Providing an opportunity for role reversal from one extreme to the other can also deepen the insights gained from the spectrogram.

The leader can also divide the group up into clusters of "less," "moderately," and "quite experienced" members and have each cluster brainstorm and present to the group as a whole any ideas they have discovered about what they bring to the group, what challenges they may have to overcome to participate fully and fairly, and what they need from other members.

By working openly with the issues as well as finding strategies for each member to share their experiences in ways that serve the group (e.g. a member with dance experience could lead a physical warm-up) the leader(s) can work with the "talents" of the "experienced actors" in ways that integrate instead of isolate other members.

Awareness of the needs of a particular grouping of young people is important for the group leader. There are also special kinds of settings within which groups may occur that carry their own challenges and conditions.

Working in special settings and situations

Action groups require privacy: a space within which members can feel safe to explore. It is also important for meetings to occur in a space in which any noise generated by the group will not be disturbing other work going on in the surrounding environment. There needs to be enough room to move, at least a bit. Other than that, most any setting will do. The nature of the setting within which groups happen, however, as well as logistical considerations, can have big effects on the progress of the work and may require adaptation of activities or readjustment of goals. In exploring these considerations, the focus will be more on clinical considerations and logistical needs and less on action strategies themselves.

Groups with single leaders

Although it will always remain my recommendation to conduct action groups for adolescents with at least two leaders, even if one is an intern or trainee, the realities of human service agencies and practices may make this impossible. There are a number of concerns that a single leader should keep in mind.

BUILDING COMPETENCE, CONFIDENCE, AND TRUST

The solo leader must pay particular attention to building the competence of the group members in utilizing the action methodologies, as well as confidence and trust in the leader and each other, before getting too deeply into the issues. Action can move group members very quickly into a depth of experience that may be beyond the group's or the leader's ability to handle until a strong foundation of skill has been developed. Working clearly with the group on boundary issues, as described earlier, can both help keep an appropriate focus and allow self-disclosure to evolve as the group gradually develops the skill to deal with it. Attending to safety issues and clear norms supports the development of confidence and trust.

It does not necessarily take longer for these attributes to develop with a solo leader, but during times of intensity or shakiness, the individual leader does not have the support provided by a leadership team. It is more difficult, therefore, when a leader works solo, to compensate for and contain disturbances and disruptions that can result from moving too quickly into deeply personal material.

DEVELOPING LEADERSHIP WITHIN THE GROUP

Out of both necessity and good group practice, with more experienced groups, or more mature group members, the single leader may call upon members to move into some supportive leadership roles, such as timekeeping, attendance, or note taking (notating issues that arise during the session). These roles can be rotated and time may be spent teaching the parameters of the roles to the members. In any group setting, the more the group accepts responsibility for itself, the more the members are likely to get from the experience. With a single leader, members sharing leadership roles provides some of the benefits of a leadership team while supporting the members to grow in confidence and interpersonal skills.

CONCRETIZING "NEGATIVE" ROLES

When there are no adult leaders to hold the "negative" roles in a drama, and certainly sometimes even when adults are present, it is generally better to use inanimate objects for such roles. In most cases, a single leader of a group should not take on any role in a psychodrama, particularly one that has a lot of "charge." Generally, the leader should explain to the group that there are some roles that hold a lot of negative energy or toward which members might need to direct very strong feelings. In these cases, the group will benefit more from using a chair or an object to play that "role." I have made good use over the years of a dressmaker's dummy, attired in female garb on one side and male on the other, for holding a wide variety of roles during dramatic enactment.

However, there could be a case in which a particular group member would clinically benefit from holding such a role. An example might be a member who is withdrawn and shy and for whom enacting a "bully" or "harasser" role might provide some role training in becoming more assertive or powerful.

The leader's task, in either case, is to make sure that every member is safe and secure during the drama. In addition, if a member is allowed to play a "negative" role, care must be taken to provide adequate de-roling for that group member so that they can put aside the negative parts of the role and so that the group will not attach these negative aspects to the person. (See Appendix D for de-roling activities.)

MAINTAINING A SHIFTING FOCUS IN GROUP SESSIONS

When working in action, it is easy for the leader to develop a strong focus on the center of the action in a sociodrama or on the protagonist in a psychodrama. It is important that the single leader keeps his or her focus moving out into the group from time to time to check in on how members are responding to the action. It may be necessary to stop the action to address things that are happening elsewhere in the space. Even with a team of adult co-leaders, the director needs to maintain a multiple focus. However, experienced members or co-leaders can help bring attention to group issues if the director is focused on the protagonist. A solo leader must utilize narrow and wide perspectives on his or her own.

DEVELOPING CLEAR NORMS FOR STOPPING THE ACTION

In developing group norms, the single leader should pay particular attention to discussion about and establishment of norms concerning how situations will be handled in which someone becomes "overwhelmed" by their own or another person's work. Group members need to know that it is better to ask for the action to stop if they become too flooded by their affect, especially during another person's work, rather than to run out of the room. Members also need to be told that if a drama in which they are protagonist becomes too intense for another member, they (the protagonists) are not to blame or at fault, and stopping the drama is not an indication that they did something wrong.

If a member leaves while the group is in session, and the leader has no co-leader, either the departing individual or the group is left alone. Neither of these outcomes is desirable.

In the event that the action is stopped, and one individual needs support, it generally should happen in the presence of the group. If this feels too intrusive, other members might be asked to pair up and talk about how they are feeling in the moment, while the leader supports the overwhelmed member more privately. Then all members can come together to share feelings about the process of operating a group safely. If the member who needed the stop in action is not the protagonist, care must be given to allow the protagonist to express his or her feelings to the group as well.

In many ways, the *process* of the group is the primary outcome, and members can be supported to observe ways in which reflecting on their process in times of difficulty serves them just as much as the work they may do in action. When possible, the group may return to the action that was occurring prior to the pause, after checking in with all members to see if they feel able to revisit the material. Otherwise, there can be an agreement to revisit it another time, if appropriate. The final decision may not please everyone, and the discomfort or displeasure then becomes "grist for the mill."

Realities of therapeutic environments may dictate the need for single leadership, despite the fact that it is not the most appropriate way to operate with adolescent groups. Whether operating as an individual, a pair, or a team, group leaders need to have a broad range of training, experience, and skills, and be "multiple role players." When operating solo, the leader is under greater pressure to have all roles functional at all times. Regular and adequate clinical supervision for solo leaders is a necessity, and one all leaders should have access to and fully utilize.

Groups with fluctuating membership

Working with a group whose membership changes from session to session presents additional unique challenges and limits the possibilities for what can be accomplished in each session and over time. This does not mean that important work cannot be done. Indeed, using action methods will likely result in being able to accomplish more in the same amount of time. Goals and procedures, however, need to be realistic and developed with awareness.

Part of the training and functioning of the group should be in supporting the more long-term members of the group in serving as "mentors" to the newer members. "Oldtimers" can be asked to share norms and procedures with the "newcomers" instead of having the leader always handle this task. This delegation of the tasks of welcoming and integrating new members helps to build interpersonal bridges as well as making the process more interesting for the returning members, who may have heard this material time and again. The realization that they are being of service to others and of value to the group can be an extremely therapeutic experience for these "helpers," while providing them with an opportunity to test and evaluate their own progress in the group.

It is also important to keep the focus of the group clear and relatively simple: something that can stand alone in one session. Unless the group is one that only occasionally fluctuates, for example, inpatient units in which members remain for

90 days with a new member introduced from time to time, it is difficult to carry over an issue or activity from one group session to the next. Some group members are likely to arrive late from their psychiatrist's appointment or have to leave early to attend a family meeting. The focus could be something that came up at that morning's "community meeting," or something that is currently on the minds of group members, such as a stressful local event. One can also use single session time to build strengths and conduct role training for healthy behavioral choices. Even if there is a sequence to these activities, they can be structured in a manner that allows each to stand alone as a distinct piece of work.

Inpatient and "locked" facilities

Inpatient facilities present their own unique challenges, especially if they are a "locked" facility or a site of incarceration. Issues of single leadership and fluctuating membership are likely to be at play in addition to the confining conditions of the environment.

Inpatient and locked facilities often operate on a behavioral model with a point system for earning levels of privileges. These systems generally focus on managing and containing behavior. If group members are encouraged to participate in more expansive and expressive activities, time may be needed at the end of sessions to cool down and refocus into a mode of behavior that won't get participants in trouble with (and the leader cursed at by) the other staff who have to deal with the "expanded" affect with which the members may leave the group. (See Appendix D for cool-down activities.)

It is helpful in these settings to communicate with other staff, since they may be impacted by the behavior of group members after group sessions. The group leader should let other staff know about the modalities being used and their possible impact, perhaps by offering an inservice training. Ideas can be solicited from the other staff about specific skills that might be the focus of some group sessions. Since many of these facilities operate on a "therapeutic community" model, the more the group goals and objectives relate to the community, the more likely the group is to operate successfully within the community as well as to address needs of the individual members.

In-school groups

Group leaders must be extremely mindful if conducting groups in a school setting. They must be conversant with school district policies and procedures as well as with the norms of the building within which they work. If the leaders are school guidance counselors, they will be familiar with the above considerations and can find "action" groups effective and appropriate for many needs.

EDUCATIONAL/SKILLS BUILDING GROUPS

Even if the group is focused on education, for example, teaching anger management skills, conflict resolution, or HIV prevention, the group leader should be aware that working in action can quickly connect participants to feelings and personal material. Students may disclose inappropriately or bring up personal matters that need follow-up that falls outside the group leader's or even the guidance counselor's purview. It may be appropriate to stop a student from disclosing further in a group and to set up an individual appointment or referral. Additionally, confidentiality is quite difficult to maintain in these kinds of groups, so norms around personal disclosure should be clear. Students can be encouraged to ask questions in the hypothetical and not use names, but to share information about the experiences of "someone they know."

In groups of this kind, therefore, the focus should be on using action to explore the issue, motivate students to learn more, and practice skills for healthy social interaction. There are many fine curricula on the market that use role playing to work with these kinds of issues. Additional tips for putting issues into action can be found in *ACTING OUT: The Workbook* (Cossa *et al.* 1996).

SUPPORT GROUPS

School counselors may desire to run groups for students dealing with common issues, such as: divorced or divorcing parents; coping with ADHD; or being gay, lesbian, etc. Action approaches can help students express feelings and frustrations as well as help develop skills for dealing constructively with life situations.

Such counseling or support groups, however, even if not strictly "therapy groups," may require signed consent by parents for members to participate if members are under the legal age. This could be a concern for non-mainstream young people who may not be ready to "come out" to parents. After checking the school policy, the counselor should inform prospective members of the policy so they will be able to make an informed decision about participating before contact is made with the parent(s) or guardian(s).

When appropriate to involve parents, information sessions, such as the kind described in Chapter 5, allow questions to be answered and consent forms to be signed. Such a session can also provide parents and guardians with ideas about what they can be doing when the teen is at home to support the work of the group. The session can also offer an opportunity for parents to set up a support network for parents of children dealing with common issues.

School counseling presents a wide range of challenges in terms of numbers of students for whom the counselor is responsible, as well as of conflicting messages about what the counselor's job is and is not. Action groups, when designed and implemented with thoughtfulness, can help maximize the use of the counselor's time and provide significant benefit to the participants.

On the other hand, community-based workers operating in school settings may have more or less leeway in terms of content areas that can be covered, but care must be taken to have a clear agreement with the school prior to the start of groups. These "outside leaders" also need to consider whether or not parental consent may be required for participation.

Nonclinical settings

Although the primary focus of this book is on the uses of action techniques in clinical settings, many of the ideas and suggestions in this book can also be employed by people leading youth groups as part of after-school programs sponsored by churches or community organizations, summer camps, or other similar programs. Sociodrama and role training can be extremely effective educational tools, and they are also likely to stir up "real" issues for participants. Group leaders in these settings must be thoughtful about the limits and boundaries of their programs and must know appropriate referral sources in the community. If issues arise for individuals within the group that go beyond the educational or social skills building goals of the program, an appropriate referral should be made.

Summary

Just as working with adolescents has challenges and rewards that are different from working with adults, so does each different type of population or setting call for different structures and a different awareness about needs and norms. The group leader has a responsibility to consider the special circumstances, and to discover the ways in which action approaches can help the work. Conversations with other professionals who are experienced with the population in question can support a group leader to become appropriately prepared for moving into a new area of endeavor.

There is, unfortunately, a significant gap between "the ideal program for young people" and the realities of human service work. Youth workers with experience in providing services to any of the populations discussed in this chapter generally have a list of frustrations at least as long as their list of success stories. However, unless we focus on the ideal and look for ways to be guided by it, in the midst of dealing with reality, we increase the probability of group leader burnout.

In the final chapter of this book, I explore some ideas for putting it all together: the theory and philosophy of Part I, the practical suggestions in Part II, the needs of special populations and settings, and the considerations for working with the changing needs of adolescents.

CHAPTER 10

Practical Considerations for Developing and Implementing Adolescent Action Groups

In 1991, the book *Psychodrama: Inspiration and Technique*, edited by Paul Holmes and Marcia Karp, offered a wide range and rich array of ideas, from a number of authors, about working psychodramatically. For me, however, the true genius of the book was in its title. It captures the magical blend of practice and theory, rational thought and spontaneity, art and science, which make psychodrama and the other expressive therapies such powerful tools for healing.

In this final chapter, I review the importance of consciously integrating philosophy, theory, and practice, the inspiration and the technique. Considerations are then offered for grounding programs in the realities of the communities in which they operate as well as in the unique reality of adolescent groups.

This book is intended more as a toolbox than a recipe book. Tools must be selected because they are suitable for the task at hand. It is true we can use a hammer to force a screw into a board, but a screwdriver works better. Here are some suggestions for ways to organize your thinking as you select the right tools.

Importance of integrating theory and philosophy with practice

My introduction to expressive therapies came from the "practice" end, with the discovery of the therapeutic nature of work I had been doing with young people in the performing arts, particularly theatre. I had a good intuitive sense about what I was doing and some background in counseling psychology, but knew that I needed to ground my work in sound theory in order to be both responsible and most effective. I also came to see the importance of having a clearly articulated philosophy of practice.

It is the philosophy of J.L. Moreno that serves as the foundation for the practice of his techniques of sociometry, psychodrama, and sociodrama. Our philosophical beliefs, as well as the theoretical foundations developed during our training and to which we subscribe, inform our practice of expressive therapies and action techniques. Conscious reflection upon one's theoretical frame and philosophical beliefs is, I believe, an essential starting point to thoughtful work as a group therapist with any age group.

Understanding theoretical and philosophical foundations

Current explorations in quantum physics, one of the most "objective" of sciences, offer the idea that we cannot measure something without affecting it, and that all we can really determine are "probabilities." A "theory" is an explanation of these probabilities: an hypothesis that attempts to make sense of information and arrange it in a form from which we can draw conclusions and create operational strategies. Theories become conserved or fixed as more people agree that these theories have something of value to offer.

As Moreno postulated in his "Canon of Creativity" (Moreno 1993, pp.17–18), the cultural conserve, at its best, warms us up to utilizing our spontaneity to engage in the creative process that allows new theories and thoughts to evolve, and new conserves to take the place of the old.

"Philosophies" are, by definition, belief systems. They provide a way to arrange our thinking to motivate our actions in a manner about which we can feel both confident and good.

No matter how utilitarian our theories, or how altruistic our philosophies may be, they are just our "best guesses" of the moment. They inform how we operate. When they remain open to evolution and development themselves, they serve us well. When they become rigid or inflexible they can hinder our work.

THEY INFLUENCE WHAT WE SEE

Some years ago, at a workshop about sexual abuse, a presenter made the statement "When all you have is a hammer, everything looks like a nail." This can be the curse of rigid theories and philosophies. They tempt us to try to fit everything we see into a framework that can be explained by what we believe to be true, for better or for worse.

One of the most remarkable training experiences I have had was while attending a workshop conducted by Rob Gordon (2001), a group psychothera-pist, at a conference in Melbourne, Australia. As the workshop progressed, Rob and I developed a strong connection. Perhaps because of this, from time to time, he would say to me, "How would you describe that?" Each time, I would express my thoughts, using psychodrama language, about a concept he had been discussing with more *analytical* language. As we participated in this process, each of our visions became fuller. Hopefully, this "verbal doubling" provided a rich experience for other workshop participants as well.

The more clearly we as group therapists can articulate our own theoretical and philosophical foundations, the more often we may: explore the ways in which they color how we view happenings within our groups; be willing to consider things from other points of view; and, become able to let go of rigid thinking, and operate instead from a place of creativity. Creative clarity both allows us to make more conscious choices about the ways we work with our groups and to approach our work with integrity as well as competence.

THEY INFLUENCE WHAT WE DO

The way we operate in a group setting is a reflection of what we believe to be *true* (at least to the extent of our best understanding of that truth in this moment) as well as of what we believe to be *right*. The most creative and therapeutic moments that I have experienced in groups over the years have not come from utilizing a technique at which I was really skillful. Rather, they have come from being present, in the moment, with my understanding and beliefs about the young people with whom I was working, and co-creating a new way of exploring the issue at hand. I also recognize, however, that other professionals, working in ways more or less differently structured from mine, could also have done equally good work.

Different approaches are better suited to different situations and populations; so are they better suited to different types of practitioners. Who we are and what we believe are part and parcel of the ways we work. As we approach our understanding of these relationships with candor, we allow ourselves to remain in a developing state, rather than falling into rigid practices.

We do not operate within a vacuum, however. Our theoretical and philosophical foundations grow out of our training environments and continue to evolve due to our group experiences. Additionally, our beliefs operate within systems that incorporate other philosophical and theoretical considerations besides our own. Below, I explore how our beliefs may be formed or changed by various systemic influences, and how these influences and/or our changing beliefs affect our professional choices.

Working within community norms

The realities of the systems within which we work must be considered in order for any programs to achieve longevity, even the most innovative and effective programs. There can exist a wide range of thoughts and beliefs within the community about how young people can best be served and what can and cannot be included in programs that serve them. Thoughtful group leaders have clear priorities, choose their "battles" wisely, and know how to compromise.

The principles that guide consensus decision making – that people work together to create solutions in which everyone gets as much of what they want as possible, and no one has to give up something essential to them – can serve to guide our learning of how to compromise as youth workers within a system that can sometimes feel oppositional or unsupportive.

A key to effective compromise in working within community systems is prioritizing the essentials: knowing what you are not willing to let go of, and what you can let go of for the moment (as difficult as it may be) if you can work toward having it later. It is possible to work in this manner without resorting to dishonesty or pretense. If youth workers openly engage in respectful dialog with the community, we can find those points upon which we all can agree. We can then use these points as the foundations of our program development. We may not be able to create our ideal program, but we can create a viable program.

As group leaders consciously examine their theoretical and philosophical principles, draw on this understanding to design program structures, and develop a clear and honest relationship with their communities, programs can be developed, implemented and grown in a manner that serves the changing needs of young people. Furthermore, they can operate with the kind of flexibility necessary to respond appropriately to the issues and events of the day as well as to the fluctuating needs of group members.

Fitting strategies to actual needs of group or population

Throughout Part II of this book, I presented action strategies that could be used to address the needs of various developmental stages of the group and of the individuals within the group. "The group" to which I was referring was hypothetical. In actual practice, and with "real" groups, action strategies must be evaluated before being used. The leader needs to consider what is actually going on for this specific group and these specific individuals at this moment in time. The printed word and the presentation of ideas through the medium of writing are intrinsically linear. Unfortunately, neither groups nor individuals develop in a linear fashion. Needs can change from session to session, or even within each session. Responsiveness to these changes is incumbent upon the leader.

Nonlinear nature of group and individual development

In reality, development of individuals and groups progresses in a staggered fashion: several steps forward then a few backward, with a total gain in the forward direction when all goes well. Stages can overlap, and groups (as well as individuals) can jump back into an earlier stage during times of stress, conflict or fear. Not only must group leaders learn to discern that these fluctuations are happening, they must also recognize them as part of the process and therefore be committed to and skilled in exploring the group dynamics that initiate movement in all directions.

PROGRESSION AND REGRESSION

I have worked with groups occasionally that progressed fairly regularly through the various stages of group development. There were, of course, the "in-between" moments during which one stage was transforming into the other, but the movement was mostly in one direction. Those groups were the exception rather than the norm. In fact this type of group development most often happened with a relatively stable group membership, comprised of ongoing participants with whom I had been working over a number of years.

There are a number of factors that can initiate a group's regression to an earlier stage. I shall discuss two here: changing membership, and stress within the group.

Changing membership

When members leave and/or new members enter, a group can regress to an earlier stage of development, and rightly so. The factors that contributed to safety have shifted and group cohesion needs to be rebuilt. I remember one group that had moved into the working stage but had lost a number of members for various reasons during its first three months. The group was slipping a bit back into transition stage, and was fairly self-aware of the movement and the cause. The group and leaders together decided to accept a number of new members after a holiday break, from a waiting list to join the group.

The decision was a good one for the overall health of the group. However, it did result in a mixed warm-up for the group, as about as many new members joined as there were members continuing. The new members entered happily and solidly engaged in beginning group behaviors. The continuing members were somewhat regressed back from working stage, but not quite all the way back to transition behaviors. Once the continuing members became more comfortable, they moved back into working mode as the new members moved into transition behaviors. It was a bit of a see-saw for a few weeks, but the continuing members were able to support the newer members and all were supported by the leaders. Gradually, all the members became a united, working group.

Stress within the group

When groups experience situations of stress, anxiety tends to increase and spontaneity tends to decrease. Stress can be caused by conflict among members, perhaps from an issue that originated outside the group and is carried in. Alternately, stress can be related to reaching a new level of trust and having deeper issues emerge. Stress can also result from a leader's poor handling of an intense situation or conflict between the leader and a member. Whatever the specific cause, the behaviors that result from the group's reaction to stress are a signal that something is amiss and needs to be addressed openly and honestly.

It is important for leaders to deal with their own reactions to stress within the group *outside* of the group, such as in team meetings with co-leaders or in supervision. To paraphrase Rudyard Kipling: If you can keep your head while the group members are losing theirs, you can help create a safe container within which the stressful events and the reaction to them can be examined and dealt with in a productive manner.

Group leaders who can identify and work with the various fluctuations that occur as an intrinsic part of the group process are likely to achieve an overall "progression" despite the occasional "regression." In addition to the more major fluctuations, however, leaders must also learn to recognize the smaller ups and downs that occur from session to session, or even within a single session. Leaders must first evaluate whether each session or activity is moving into a more *contracted* or *explosive* space, and therefore determine whether *expansion* or *containment* is required.

EXPANSION AND CONTAINMENT

I first encountered some of the basic concepts expressed in this section, and the terminology used to express them, in an article by Renée Emunah (1990).

Adolescents, in groups and individually, by nature of their changing physiology as well as environmental factors, naturally experience swings in affect. Sometimes, members can be very contracted and withdrawn and difficult to get into action. Other times, the energy of the group is explosive and "all over the place," difficult to focus.

Some action techniques are expansive, others are containing. Some can be either, depending on how they are used. Leaders should consider both the energy of the group and its degree of warm-up in deciding which activities to use in a given session. One might choose expansive activities to help a group move out of a contracted state, or choose containing activities if a group is explosive. Paradoxically, leaders might choose to help a group move through one state or another by exaggerating its nature: becoming even more contracted and feeling most fully the restricted nature of this condition, or allowing members to explode and "blow off steam" in a safe way. The choice may vary with the goals the leader has for the session, as well as the leader's available patience on a given day, but the choice should be a conscious one. Following are a sampling of activities and how they can be employed to expand or contain the energy of a group.

Graphic arts

Graphic arts, such as drawing, collage, or sculpting, are containing in nature. They provide a conveniently bounded container, the piece of paper or lump of clay, within which excess energy can be focused. For a group of pre and early teens whose leaders I was supervising, and who arrived at group directly from school with their energies scattered, a nonstructured art activity was available when they arrived for each session. It served as a transition from the energy of the day into the focused attention of the group.

Because of their containing nature, graphic arts can also be used when a group has very low energy as a way of respecting where members are in the moment. Utilizing an art project can help members get some energy out and into exploration of issues without making demands on the members for a lot of physical activity or emotional displays.

Movement

Movement activities can be used either to expand or contain. A physical warm-up activity can meet the group at its level of energy and gradually move it in either direction. It can begin very low key, for example, and gradually build in intensity, or vice versa.

When a group is feeling stuck and contracted, a movement activity can be designed to exaggerate the "stuckness," encouraging members to become even more contracted and stuck to the point of discomfort. A spontaneous release into a more expanded state will generally follow, merely from the need of the body to let go of the extreme tension created. Similarly, a group can be directed in very energetic (though safely contained) movement as a way to burn up some of the excess energy before bringing the members to a more focused place.

Challenge games

Challenge games, such as Group Juggle, described in Chapter 5, can also be used to build energy or meet the energy of the group and help to focus it. Because its challenge can be framed in several ways, for example, how many objects can be managed by the group without dropping, or how quickly can we complete the series of passes with three objects, leaders can structure this activity to serve the needs of the moment.

Games with highly physical challenges that require thought as well are good for groups whose energy is high. Games that require thought first, and then action arising from a plan, serve the low energy group.

Multiple activities

There are times when the energy of the group is not only disjointed but also varied. Some members may be "bouncing off the walls" while others are lethargic. Offering the option for several activities to happen at once allows each member to be met "where they are" and, hopefully, come to a common place after a time. Even in the single leader group, an art area can be set up that requires minimal supervision while the leader focuses on those members whose energy is high and needs containing. The example given in Chapter 6 of non-directed activity leading to playing house, is a vivid illustration of employing multiple activities.

Dramatic warm-up

Simple dramatic warm-up activities, especially those that can be done sitting, work well for building the energy of a lethargic group. Using an activity such as Parent/Kid Scenes (Chapter 5), with the instruction that each scene is about something that parents and kids fight about, will generally engage most group members and build the energy fairly quickly.

Dramatic enactment

Dramatic enactment is almost always expansive. If moving into sociodrama, psychodrama, or drama therapy activity with a very high energy group, creating a few scenes in slow motion may help to contain energy to a constructive level. One can also use theatre activities that require thought, such as asking each person who initiates a new sentence to begin with a successive letter of the alphabet.

If the group is beginning from a fairly low energy place, using a dramatic warm-up first helps build the energy necessary for more indepth work.

Although not exhaustive by any means, these examples provide a sense of how activities can be consciously applied for the purposes of expansion or containment. The inexperienced leader can too easily be caught unawares when trying out a new activity, unless thought is given to activity selection from these perspectives. Leaders can, as part of the group norm setting, work with the group to create and practice agreed upon signals for containment, such as saying "Pause the action," or blinking the lights. In this manner expansive (and noisy) activities, inevitable at some points in an action group, can be stopped, slowed down, quieted down in an instant as part of the normal process, rather than as a struggle for control.

In working with adolescent groups, fluctuations of energy, affect, and ability to focus are par for the course. Group leaders who cannot change gears rather quickly are probably not suited to action groups with young people. Working with the energy of the group and refocusing it work much better than fighting the energy of the group and demanding that members behave differently. All of these elements discussed in this chapter are part of what the group leader must learn to juggle.

For group leaders, it may seem at times as though the amount of information that needs to be understood and the number of factors that need to be managed are overwhelming. The more one can get in touch with these feelings of being overwhelmed by the process, and the more one can observe how these feelings change with experience, the better one can understand the developmental continuum of the adolescent experience. Young people also move through periods of being overwhelmed with the complexities of negotiating an adult world and can, with experience, develop the needed awareness and skills to negotiate successfully.

Summary

The quest to be an effective group leader for adolescents is a noble and complex one. It is also a very personal one, both in terms of the reasons we choose to work with this population as well as how we do it. Leaders must have a good understanding of their own theoretical and philosophical foundations, and recognize the ways in which those foundations affect how they view what is happening in groups as well as how they respond to it. The successful application of action techniques requires an integration of the theoretical and the practical.

Group leaders must also recognize that they operate within a community in which needs, expectations, and norms of the various elements may not always be complementary. Holding true to their commitment to the young people they serve, group leaders must also learn to prioritize and compromise for their programs to survive.

Group leaders, like jugglers, keep many things moving at the same time and must learn to respond to the changing needs of their groups. Group and individual development are nonlinear, and leaders need to recognize and work comfortably with the progressions and regressions, expansions and contractions that are an integral part of the adolescent group.

Finally, group leaders must recognize that adolescence does not arrive full blown and depart in a single moment. Adolescence is a continuum of experiences in which young people develop in many interacting and often conflicting ways at the same time. The effective group leader, like the wilderness guide, can help young people negotiate the dangerous territory, enjoy the breathtaking scenery, and arrive in their "new land" more ready to create the future.

Sample Information Pack
for Participants and Families

_____ offers a voluntary program for young people aged _____, which runs from _____, through _____. _____ groups use expressive arts group therapy to provide support to members for positive change and growth. The following pages offer a statement of the workings of the program.

Groups meet _____ on _____ from _____ to _____. There are no sessions _____. Special activities may, however, be scheduled during these times for those who are available. Sessions may or may not be held on other school holidays.

The program utilizes expressive arts group therapy to help members better understand who they are, gain support, develop a more positive self-image, and explore options. Theater activities are used as a means of expressing and sharing.

Some thoughts on therapy

Psychotherapy, from its Greek root, means "healing the soul." All of us carry with us the hurts and confusions of a lifetime. The group process helps us to see that we are not alone, and that, with support, our lives can be different. What is sometimes true for people involved in a group therapy experience is that feelings not often looked at may be stirred up. This occasionally can lead to feeling anxious or depressed. We acknowledge these reactions as being normal, and provide the means to deal with these feelings within the group setting.

_____ works through group process. Although leaders are available to answer questions and offer support to individual members, they do not provide individual counseling. In the event that a participant is in need of individual counseling on a regular basis, the leaders can make a referral to an appropriate counselor in the school or community. This process requires parental consent and cooperation. It is not in the best interest of the participant to be counseled individually by one of the group leaders, as there would likely be problems with confidentiality and role confusion.

If students experience difficulty with other members of the group, they are encouraged to use the group as a means of working it out. Leaders offer support to those who find it difficult to start this process, but do not work with students apart from the group in ironing out difficulties. Any issues raised about members by other participants cannot be "held in secret" by the group leaders.

Family contact

Support from parents is important to a participant's success in the program. We must clarify, however, that this is not a family counseling program. The program is designed to serve the participants.

As youth work in the program, it is possible that behaviors will start to change, at home and elsewhere. Sometimes even a positive change in behavior can seem unsettling to a family that has become accustomed to a particular way of operating. Should a parent/guardian have a concern about their child that they wish to bring to the attention of the group leaders, the content of the communication will be shared with that participant. If it is necessary for the group leaders to meet with parents, the group member must be present. In the event that a family feels it needs assistance in working through difficulties it is experiencing, the leaders will make a referral to an appropriate community agency.

Confidentiality

All personal and family information that is shared as part of this program will be kept strictly confidential, with a few exceptions as are stated in the authorization forms we ask participants and parents/guardians to sign. Program leaders are bound by law to report any instances or clear suspicions of physical abuse, sexual abuse, or neglect. If a participant seems actively suicidal, or has indicated an intention to cause harm to another, these must also be reported. With these exceptions, what is said or done within the group remains within the group.

_____ group leaders do not initiate communication with school authorities, other counselors, public officials, etc., except at the request of the participant. Should we be contacted by any outside person or agency about a member, the content of the communication will be shared with the member.

Input from parents, schools, etc.

We value the insight that parents, teachers, etc. have about the young people who will be participating in our program. We feel that it is important for participants to understand that their actions and behaviors have an effect on others and color the way they are perceived by others. It is also important for students to receive feedback from their families and communities, from their group leaders, and from each other in evaluating their progress within the program. We encourage students to seek this kind of feedback. _____ staff do not seek this kind of feedback about our members except by means of a parent feedback questionnaire at year's end.

Intake and selection process

The intake process begins with potential members and parent(s)/guardian(s) attending an Information Session to understand the program better and to have questions answered. If the youth is interested, and the parent(s) are in agreement, the potential member is invited to attend some introductory group meetings to find out more about the process before making a commitment. For students under 18 years of age, parental consent is required for participation in the program. After the introductory sessions, those students who are still interested in the program, and willing to make a commitment to the time and effort expected of them, will be eligible for selection.

We are limited in the number of students we can accept into the program. We try to maintain a good representation of gender, age, and life experience of our students. Our program is designed for those who can benefit by what we have to offer. Since we may not be able to accept all who apply, we will encourage those students not selected to apply again next year. We do maintain a waiting list in the event that places open up during the year.

Program participation

Once members begin the program, the leaders reserve the right to ask them to leave the program if: they are unable to follow established norms; they do not maintain regular attendance; or they cause severe disruption to the group. No one will be asked to leave without prior discussion with the leaders. Should a member consider withdrawing from the program at any time, it is requested that they discuss their concerns with the leaders and the group.

It will be the responsibility of the members to arrange transportation to and from all regularly scheduled meetings. Staff cannot provide rides home after meetings or activities.

Program norms and guidelines

The norms and guidelines established for _____ are attached.

Cost

[Note: Your policy and procedures about cost should go here.]

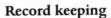

Record keeping

Agency policy requires that we maintain statistical records of the impact of the program on its members. We use a combination of approaches, which will allow staff and members to develop goals and chart their progress. All member files are strictly confidential. The members and staff of _____ are the only ones who have access to this information. Reporting to our funding sources is done only in terms of numbers and demographic information (age, gender, location, etc.).

Sample Intake and Permission Forms

Application/intake form

Full name: _____ Age: _____

Date of birth: _____ Phone: _____

Address: _____ City: _____

_____

_____

State: _____ Postal code: _____ E-mail: _____

School: _____ Grade: _____

School contact or guidance person: _____

Parent/guardian information

Mother:_____Father: _____

Address: _____

_____

_____

Phone (H): _____

(W): _____

(M): _____

Appendix B is reproduced here with the permission of Monadnock Family Services who is not in any way representing or warranting the suitability of these forms for anyone's use.

I heard about the program from: _____

I am interested in participating because: _____

In case of emergency, and parents are not contactable, please notify

Name: _____ Phone: _____

Family doctor: _____ Phone: _____

Address: _____

_____

Any regular medications?

_____

_____

Any physical limitations?

_____

_____

Others residing in household with youth and parent(s):

Name: _____ Age: _____ Relationship: _____

The following information is used for statistical purposes only and is optional. It is, of course, confidential.

Any special educational coding? _____

Any grades failed? _____ Which? _____

Has the youth ever been involved with juvenile court?_____

Current counseling, youth? _____ Family? _____

Previous counseling, youth? _____ Family?_____

Other information that might help staff to serve the member better

_____

_____

_____

Authorization for participation

Re: _____ Date of birth: _____

I,_____, give permission for my child to participate in the following group(s) for the _____ program year, as described in the information sheet for members and parents.

I understand that all personal and family data will be kept strictly confidential. I also understand that program staff are required by law to report any suspected cases of physical or sexual abuse, neglect, and intention to commit suicide or to cause physical harm to another.

I agree I will not withhold permission for my child to participate in the program as a consequence of behavior at home or in school.

This authorization expires at the conclusion of the program year, _____, or at the end of my child's participation, whichever occurs first.

_____   _____
Participant's signature   Parent/guardian signature

                                                          Date:_____

Sample Group Norms

Confidentiality

- All material discussed in group stays in group. This applies to group members and group leaders alike.

- Group leaders are required by law to report cases of suspected physical and sexual abuse, and serious intention to injure self or others. If reporting is necessary, group leaders will work with the member to decide how to proceed.

- Group leaders do not initiate communication about a group member with parents, school officials, or anyone outside the group except at the request, and if possible, in the presence, of a group member.

- If group leaders are contacted by an outside person or agency regarding a member, the content of that communication is shared with the member, privately, and the member will be encouraged to share this information with the group.

- Any information brought to group leaders by a member about another member cannot be held in secret from the member by the leaders.

Respect

- The group is a safe place to express feelings, thoughts, and ideas. Members respect one another's right to be who they are without fear of ridicule.

Appendix C is reproduced here with the permission of Monadnock Family Services who is not in any way representing or warranting the suitability of these forms for anyone's use.

- No form of verbal or physical abuse, or threats of violence against another will be permitted at any time.
- Members are encouraged to use physical contact with each other consciously and kindly.
- Excessive profanity is not an acceptable form of group behavior or communication.
- Members will not attend sessions under the influence of alcohol or illegal drugs. State and federal laws have made it illegal for people under the age of 18 to purchase, possess, or use tobacco products. All members are discouraged from using tobacco products during group activities.
- Members of the group will respect the space in which the group interacts, and will observe the rules of those facilities within which we work.

Participation

- Each member is encouraged to participate in all activities of the group. The choice to do so remains the member's.
- Members are encouraged to reveal personal material to the group when they choose, and to the extent that this is appropriate to their needs.
- Success of the program and its benefits to members depend on each member's full, regular, and punctual participation.
- Any pattern of absence or tardiness by a member will result in review of their member status by the leaders and the group members.
- In the event of illness or emergency, members should notify group leaders as soon as the member is aware of the need to miss a meeting. Messages may be sent through other members, if necessary.

Relationships between members

- Members are strongly discouraged from becoming "romantically" involved with each other, both during and outside of group activities.
- The group is not an appropriate place for "dating" behaviors.
- Members pursuing friendships with other members outside the group will keep the confidentiality norm in mind at all times.
- Members are reminded that paired relationships may limit their capacities to be fully and equally present for all members of the group.

Termination

- Leaders reserve the right to ask a member to leave the group, for a session or permanently, if he or she: does not follow these established norms; does not maintain regular attendance; causes severe disruption to the group.

- No one will be asked to leave without having the opportunity to have a discussion with the leaders and the group about this request.

- Should a member consider withdrawing from the program at any time, they are requested to discuss their concerns, and/or to say good-byes, with the leaders and the group.

Other Ideas for Opening and Closing Circles, Warm-ups, Cool-downs, and De-roling

Opening and Closing Circles

Opening and Closing Circles are one way to mark the beginning and ending of a group session. Opening Circles help members to bring their focus clearly to the group and to share something about themselves or to warm up to issues or themes for the session. Closing Circles allow members to end as a group and may help them reflect on the session, set goals for the time between sessions, or ground more fully in the present if the session was a particularly intense one. For the purposes of this listing, suggestions are grouped according to where they might be used in the development of the group.

Group interviews and/or initial sessions

OPENING CIRCLES

Opening Circles at this stage of group development should always begin with members stating their names before completing the question or action for the day.

1. Stand up, say your name and make a gesture about how you feel today. The group will echo and mirror back to you both your name and your gesture.

2. State your name and one reason you considered/are considering joining this group.

3. State your name and share one activity that you like to do.

4. State your name and one personal fact you'd like to share.

5. State your name and complete the sentence "I came today because..."

6.   State your name and complete the sentence "What I would like to have happen today is..."

7.   State your name and share a favorite television character/show.

8.   State your name and share your favorite flavor of ice cream.

9.   State your name and share your favorite/least favorite school subject.

10. State your name and mime what you look like when you first wake up in the morning.

CLOSING CIRCLES

1.   Describe your experience of this group session in a word or phrase.

2.   Describe how you feel right now with a word or a phrase.

3.   Use a sound and movement or gesture to share how you feel right now.

4.   Name one thing you enjoyed about today's group.

5.   Finish the sentence, "The moral of today's group is..."

6.   Give one reason you are planning to come back to this group.

7.   Name one activity you did today that was difficult for you.

8.   If this group were a movie, what would you name it?

9.   State in one sentence how it feels to be a member of this group at this point.

10. What is one thing you hope to gain from participating in this group?

Sessions early in the group experience

OPENING CIRCLES

Opening Circles at this stage of group development may still begin with members stating their names as an aid to everyone's learning names, especially if some new members entered after the group started.

1.   Share a special object you brought from home and describe the reasons it is important to you. If you forgot to bring one, share what you would have brought.

2.   Share an adjective that you think describes you.

3.   Share how you think you tend to act in new situations.

4.   Share one thing to which you can give 100 percent attention.

5. Name a character in a book, movie, or television show with whom you identify.

6. Name one goal you would like to accomplish while being a member of this group.

7. Name one thing that you think will help the group feel safe and comfortable together.

8. Share one fact that people in the group probably don't know about you that you want to share.

9. Share what it is about the group that has kept you coming back.

10. Share what you think is the most important group norm and why.

CLOSING CIRCLES

1. Name one thing you are looking forward to before the next meeting.

2. Make a sound that describes how you are feeling right now.

3. Name a time during the group when you lost/kept focus and say why and how.

4. Share something you'd like to accomplish/change for yourself with the group's support.

5. Share one way you are feeling differently at the end of group than you were at the start of group.

6. What is one thing you are taking from today's group that might be useful in the coming week?

7. If today's group were a type of music, what would it be?

8. Share something positive that you noticed about another group member today.

9. Describe today's group meeting in three words.

10. On a scale of one to ten, how focused were you at today's group session?

Sessions in the middle of the group experience
OPENING CIRCLES

1. State a topic or issue that is important to you for whatever reason.

2. Give a word, phrase, face, or a sound of how you feel right now.

3. What is one thing that stands out for you about the last group session?

4.   Complete the sentence, "Something I'd like to change about myself is..."

5.   If you were writing a play about the state of the world, what would the title be?

6.   If you were writing a play about your life, what would the title be?

7.   Ask an interesting question to the person on your right.

8.   Make up your own Opening Circle question, and answer it.

9.   What is one way you are different now than you were a year ago?

10.   Name three "roles" you play in group or life.

CLOSING CIRCLES

1.   Describe a personal goal for the coming week.

2.   Name one person you can count on for support.

3.   If you were giving yourself a report card for how well you participated in group today, what would be written in the section "other comments?"

4.   If you were grading the whole group today for how well members worked together, what grade would you give?

5.   What is one thing you feel is your responsibility as a group member?

6.   Name a goal for yourself that you want to focus on in group in the coming sessions.

7.   Name an obstacle you've overcome in your life and something you learned from the experience.

8.   Name a quality about yourself that you have become more aware of while participating in this group.

9.   If today were the final session of group, what is one thing you would regret not having accomplished?

10.   What is one way you are going to be good to yourself in the coming week?

Sessions during the later part of the group experience
OPENING CIRCLES

1.   Complete the sentence, "So far in this group I have been..."

2.   Complete the sentence, "Before this group is over, I would like..."

3.   What is something that gets in the way of your saying what you feel and need?

4.   Use a puppet to tell the group something about you that they don't already know that you are ready to share.

5.   How can the group support you in reaching your goals by the end of the sessions?

6.   Why have you remained a member of this group?

7.   State what you need to be fully present for the group today.

8.   What do you hope will be true for you ten years from now?

9.   Finish the sentence, "What I like about starting and ending group on time is…"

10.   What is really working/not working for you about the group?

CLOSING CIRCLES

1.   Name a goal you have achieved already in group.

2.   Share one way in which the group supports you in your life.

3.   State something you appreciate about the person on your right.

4.   What is one way the group is different now than when we started?

5.   What is something you can take with you from today's group?

6.   What is one piece of advice you give to others that you should take for yourself?

7.   Share one way you are different now than you were at the beginning of the group sessions.

8.   Complete the sentence, "If I were a leader of this group, I would …"

9.   What is your best memory of the group so far?

10.   What is one way you have really worked in the group so far?

Sessions as the group is nearing its end
OPENING CIRCLES

1.   What do you want/need from the final meetings of the group?

2.   What is left unsaid for you in this group?

3.   What is left undone for you in this group?

4. How have group members supported you since the start of the sessions?

5. Share a metaphor for your participation in this group.

6. If you could create a picture of what this group has meant to you, what colors would you use?

7. If they made a movie about this group, what would they name it?

8. What will you miss most about this group when it is over?

9. What will you miss least about the group?

10. How do you generally deal with endings and loss?

CLOSING CIRCLES

1. Describe your experience of this group in a word or phrase.

2. If this group were to be offered again, how should it be different?

3. What do you think would be different in your life now if you had not been in this group?

4. How would you like the ending of this group to be different for you than endings generally are?

5. What is one thing you would like to have be a part of our final group meeting?

6. Complete the sentence, "How I want to be remembered is..."

7. What are some ways you will cope with stress once the group has ended?

8. What do you take with you from the group?

9. What is something you would like to leave behind as you leave the group?

10. Complete the sentence, "If this final meeting of the group were a movie, my exit line would be..."

Warm-ups

Warm-ups stimulate discussion and help the group members get to know one another, move gradually into action, begin to explore an issue or theme, or transition from talk to action. They can build the energy for the group or help to contain it. With those that involve physical contact and activity, norms around respect and safety may need to be reviewed. For the purposes of this listing, suggestions are grouped according to where they might be used in the development of the group.

Group interviews and / or initial sessions

1. *Who started the movement?* Members stand in a circle. One person is asked to leave the room while a "leader" is selected. The leader begins a simple movement which all group members mirror. The member who left is invited back in and moves to the center of the circle. As the activity progresses the leader changes the movement and the group members mirror the change. The member in the circle tries to guess who is the leader.

2. *Building a group structure.* The group leader puts a collection of objects in the middle of the room. The group's task is to build the highest free-standing structure they can from these objects. A time limit may be set. Once completed, the height of the object is measured. Members discuss what they might do to make a taller structure and then have another go at the task. When the activity is complete, the leader facilitates a discussion of the roles that each member took during the task.

3. *Pass the mask.* Members sit in a circle. One person makes a face and turns to a person next to him or her who must mirror the face. The same face can be passed all the way around the circle, or each member can receive a face and then transform it into another one before passing it on.

4. *Counting to ten as a group.* Group members sit in a circle. The following instruction is given: "When I say 'go,' the task of the group is to count, sequentially, from one to ten. Anyone who would like to start may do so. Anyone who would like to say the next number may do so. No one can say two numbers in a row. You cannot just take turns around the circle. There can be no discussion. If two people say a number at the same time, I will say 'go' again and everything returns to the start. Go."

5. *Tag-word improvisation.* Two people begin an improvisation. It can be about anything. At any point another group member can call out a word or brief phrase that was just said by one of the actors. The action freezes. The person who called out the word replaces the actor who said it. The person going in must initiate a totally new scene, using the "tag word" in the opening line.

6. *"Tell me about the time when..."* This can be done one member at a time, or people can be paired, in which case it becomes "Tell your partner about the time when...." Either the leader or the partner ends the sentence with some improbable and/or ridiculous statement, and the person makes up a short story about the situation. Some examples are: "Tell me about the time when... the pizza from outer space kidnapped your sister; you were having brunch with the president/prime minister/etc. and you threw up

on his or her shoes; your eyebrow jumped off your face and ate your dog."

7. *Listening to the silence.* Instruct group members to sit quietly, with eyes closed, if that feels comfortable, and listen to hear how many sounds they can notice and identify in the environment. After a minute or so, share what was heard.

8. *Collective story telling.* One group member is asked to begin telling a made-up story. Each time the leader rings a bell (claps hands, says a certain word, etc.) the next person in the circle must continue the story where the last person left off, even if it is in mid-sentence.

9. *Role reversal with a character.* Each member takes a turn standing in front of an empty chair and tells the group who is in the chair. It should be a famous person from history or a character from a book or play or movie. The group member asks a question of the character, then sits in the chair and becomes the character and answers the question.

10. *"What I wish I had told you is…"* Each member takes a turn standing in front of an empty chair and *does not* tell the group who is in the chair. It should be someone in their life who they wish they had been able to say something to but didn't. As each member has the chance to say what was unsaid, she or he may or may not want to sit in the chair themselves and give a response.

Sessions early in the group experience

1. *Tense and relax.* This is a physical activity in which the leader names various body parts and group members are then alternately instructed to tense the muscles in this part, and then allow them to relax. This can build up to total body tensing and relaxing. It is a good warm-up to help get people more into their bodies in preparation for other movement activities, such as the following one.

2. *Bound/free movement.* Members are instructed to move about the space in ways that feel bound and restricted, for example, as if in chains, walking through honey, or fighting against a very strong wind. Then they are instructed to move in ways that are free, like floating or flying, or just being happy and easy-going on a warm and sunny day. Instructions can move people from one state to another. Discussion can follow about life situations that feel bound or free.

3. *Three changes.* Group members stand facing a partner and noticing all the details of the way their partner is attired. Partners then face away from each other and make three visible changes to their appearance, for

example, moving a watch from one wrist to the other, buttoning or unbuttoning something, etc. Partners then face one another and see if they can spot the changes.

4. *Rhythm circle.* Members sit in a circle. Using various percussion instruments (drums, rattles, etc.) or just hands and feet, one member begins a rhythmic pattern. One by one, other members add to the rhythm until all are participating, then members drop out one by one until the original member is left. Discussion between successive attempts can focus on what would make it "more interesting" or "work better." Processing can focus on how this rhythm circle can be a metaphor for the group experience.

5. *General mills.* Group members are instructed to "mill about in the space" without making any kind of contact or even noticing other people in the room. After a time, they are instructed to begin to be aware of others but still make no contact. Gradually, contact can be included, starting with eye contact and building up to verbal greetings, connecting in pairs, pairs connecting to each other, and so on until the entire group is physically connected.

6. *Stretch band.* Using a "stretch band," a large piece of elastic fabric that has been joined into the equivalent of a large elastic band, all members in the group stand inside the band leaning out and see if they can balance each other, notice how one person's movement affects the whole group, etc. Once "stretch band" activity begins, the group will spontaneously develop many ways to use it. A parachute activity is similar.

7. *Issue/words improvisation.* The group generates a list of possible "real-life" issues, such as substance abuse, teen pregnancy, divorce, etc., and writes them in one column of a blackboard or whiteboard. A second column is then generated of nonrelated words or phrases, the more unusual the better, such as rubber chicken or burlap underwear. A pair of group members begins a scene about any of the topics. At some point in the scene, one of the pair must find a way to work in one of the words or phrases from the list without losing the meaning of the scene. Once that task is achieved, someone from the group calls "freeze" and takes the place of one of the original pair and initiates a new scene about another of the topics on the list, in which a new word must be used.

8. *School bus.* Members are arranged as though they are sitting in pairs on a school bus. Each pair is given a number. Pairs begin conversations about any topics they wish, all going at the same time. When the leader calls a number, all other pairs freeze and the scene focuses on what is being said by that numbered pair. After a short while the leader calls, "all numbers,"

and the scene reverts to all pairs talking again until the next number is called.

9. *Family portraits.* Using other group members, each member has the opportunity to create a portrait of their family showing the relationship between members by position, posture, and gesture. A variation is for the member to give each person in the portrait a word or phrase to say in a particular sequence. The member who created the portrait looks at it from outside as well as from their place in the portrait and, if time allows, from the places of other significant family members.

10. *Portal into the future.* Using chairs or other furniture or even group members, members take turns creating their "portal into the future." Standing in the portal, they can be asked to describe it as well as be asked questions about what is on each side of it, what they need to get through the portal, what has led them to it, etc. Questions may be asked by the leader or other group members.

Sessions in the middle of the group experience

1. *Paired and group mirrors.* Members pair up and stand facing a partner. One person initiates movement and the other follows, alternating leadership until they get to the point at which they are co-creating the movement. This can be done in small groups and be built up to the creation of a group mirror activity.

2. *Movement of opposite qualities.* Group members move about the space in ways that are suggested by the leader, or group members, to explore opposites, such as passive/active, heavy/light, depressed/energized, etc. From time to time, the action can be frozen and members can share "A time I feel like this is…"

3. *Balancing bodies.* Working in pairs, group members find various ways to make contact (respectfully) and lean against each other in ways that balance. As they gain confidence, they can work on moving from one position of balance through a state of nonbalance, to find a new balance point.

4. *Animal movements.* Group members are instructed to move about the space at various speeds and with various qualities of movement. After they are loosened up a bit, they are given the instruction to imagine themselves to be an animal and let their movements evolve into the movement of that animal. Animals can encounter each other as they move about the space. After a time, members are instructed to move back into their human

movement, but to bring a quality of that animal with them into the movement.

5.   *Worst day tableaux.* Members take turns using other members to create tableaux of the worst day or worst experience that they had during the past week. The tableaux can remain silent or be given sound or words. Members see the tableaux from without as well as within.

6.   *Collage of my life.* Members have a certain amount of time to create a collage representing their lives, using words and pictures already cut from magazines, etc., and spread out on the floor or table. For sharing, each member becomes his or her collage and speaks: "I am Michael's life. Over here you see this image of a dragon; that represents…"

7.   *Role cards.* Group members are given four or five index cards and asked to write on them various roles that they or others play, including an adjective and a noun, such as the "good student," the "argumentative son," or the "angry friend." The leader(s) may also prepare some cards. All cards are then spread out on the floor and members are asked to walk around and notice which ones play a major part in their lives. They can be instructed to stand next to a role they enjoy playing, are forced into playing, hate playing, etc., and to speak from those roles.

8.   *Feeling cards.* These can be created in a similar manner to the "role cards" and placed on the floor. Members move about at random and are told to freeze and look at a nearby card and complete the sentence, "A time when I feel _____ is when…"

9.   *Concretizing ambivalence.* Members select something about which they are feeling ambivalent, pulled in two directions. Three chairs are placed side by side. Members, in their turn, begin in the center chair identifying the two opposite pulls, for example, this part of me wants to have a boyfriend or girlfriend very much, but this part of me feels that the one I have treats me very poorly. Someone is selected from the group to play the member, as the original member then demonstrates each of the voices. The member then selects group members to play these roles as the original member moves back into the center chair. This can expand from a warm-up to a full scale psychodrama with appropriate role reversal, etc.

10.   *Power continuum.* A line is made on the floor with masking tape with four or five hash marks along it at intervals. One end is marked "most powerful," and the other "least powerful." Members take turns walking the line and reflecting on times they feel "most," "quite a bit," "a bit," "not very," and "least" powerful.

Sessions during the later part of the group experience

1. *Baggage claim.* Unlike the baggage claim at an airport, in which people pick up their baggage, in this warm-up people decide what baggage they want to leave behind. It can be facilitated to be a very brief activity, a psychodramatic vignette, or even a full drama. The "baggage" may be specified or remain metaphoric.

2. *Relationships through movement.* Group members are directed to move about the room until they are asked to stop. They then pair up with another group member and explore their relationship as members of the group, through movement and sound only. If there is time, all possible pairings occur before there is any verbal discussion.

3. *Objects as self.* Members are invited to look around the room and find an object to represent themselves. It can come from sand tray figures, art supplies, etc. (An environment rich in objects is important.) Speaking as the object, they tell the group about why the person who selected it did so, and what the choice says about the person who made it.

4. *Desert island sociodrama.* As a full group, or in subgroups, members enact a drama about a group of people stranded on a desert island who are taking stock of what resources and abilities they have between them to help them survive, and which resources and abilities they will need to develop or discover. Processing can also include leadership roles that emerged at this point in the group's development and how they might be different from roles explored at the start of the group.

5. *Quadrant work.* The floor is marked by two intersecting and perpendicular lines making a four-square cross. Each line is marked with a pair of opposite qualities, such as "advance/retreat" and "direct/indirect." Group members move from quadrant to quadrant and explore, first, movements that fit the quadrant description: "direct advance," "direct retreat," etc. Then members can reflect on characters in books or movies that hold these qualities: Superman is a "direct advancer," etc. Finally, they can reflect on or create scenes about times in their lives in which they behave or act in these ways; I am an "indirect advancer" when I want to get something out of my father.

6. *Scrapbook of past, present, and future.* Group members enlist other group members to create "photographs" of what their life was like in the past, what it is like in the present, and how they would like it to be in the future.

7. *Telling secrets.* Using cushions and blankets if available, members gather on the floor, with heads facing the center of the circle and enact a "slumber

party" at which people are sharing secrets with each other. This is an opportunity to share something they have been meaning to but have yet to share.

8. *Invisible friend.* Members take turns becoming their own "invisible friend," who is interviewed about the person by the group and leader.

9. *Two scarves.* Members each select two scarves and choose one to represent something that is working in their lives and the other to represent something that they'd like to be different. From these two roles, they are interviewed about what each aspect is trying to teach the person.

10. *The gift and the mirror.* Members sit in a circle and each tells the person on the right or left of some intangible gift they would like to give to this person, for example, the ability to be more honest about how they are feeling, the ability to laugh at themselves more easily. Then members are instructed to go around the circle a second time and reflect on how the gift they gave their fellow group member is something that they need in their own lives.

Sessions as the group is nearing its end

1. *Family relationship progression sculptures.* Each member uses other group members to create two sculptures of their family: one as they were in relationship to it when the group started, and one at this point in time.

2. *Gender fishbowl.* Male members of the group sit in a large circle, while female members, in a smaller circle within the larger, discuss what it has been like to be female in a mixed gender group, and vice versa. This can be used with any different subgroupings within the full group.

3. *Mask-making series.* Using a simple technique for mask making, such as decorating a cut-out done on a paper plate, members create three self-masks: how they were when they first entered the group, how they are as they are leaving, and how they hope to be in the future.

4. *Friendship sculptures.* Working in various combinations, group members sculpt the relationships that have evolved between group members over the course of the group sessions.

5. *Children's story or fairy tale.* Group members select or make up a children's story or fairy tale to enact that is a metaphor for their experience of the group. It can be adapted as needed.

6. *Feedback posters.* Each member makes a collage or simple drawing to represent themselves. These are passed in a circle around the group, and

each member adds words or images that serve as their appreciation for and feedback to the originating member.

7.   *Highlights of the group in snapshots or scenes.* Members work together to decide on and create representations of highlights of their experiences together in the group.

8.   *Chain improvisations about endings.* Group members participate in a series of quick improvisations whose theme is endings, and the various ways that people handle them.

9.   *"As I leave the group, I am taking with me…"* Members are sitting in a circle and, as with the familiar games in which the second member repeats what the first has said and then adds to it, each member repeats what those before them have said they are taking from the group and then adds something new to the list until all have had at least one turn.

10. *Reflection in movement.* The group members stand in a cluster as the leader calls out various high and low points of the group sessions. Without thinking or discussion, members create an expression of the moment or incident given using movement and sound.

Cool-downs and de-roling

Both activities for cool-downs and for de-roling help members and the group move from a place of greater engagement and/or affect, to one of less engagement or affect. Because they may be needed and used at any point in the group and are nonspecific to developmental stage, there is no subdivision in the list of suggestions.

Cool-downs

Whenever the group has been involved in an activity or discussion with high affect, a period of cool-down is needed before members leave the group space and move out into their lives. This sometimes happens naturally if the affect-laden experience has been completed and there is ample time remaining in the group for process and discussion. If there is little time available, cool-down activities that help bring the members to a more neutral affect state can be employed. They generally bring the focus on the environment, call for members to meet a mental or physical challenge, or encourage anticipation of neutral or pleasant future events. Some examples follow.

1.   *Touch blue.* The leader names a series of criteria, and the members must find something in the room that meets each criterion, and go touch it, for example, "touch something in the room that is blue, is transparent, is the same color as your shoes." Members must touch this object with some part of their bodies.

2. *Seek and point.* The leader notices something in the room and describes it. Then, members find what the leader is describing and point to it.

3. *"Line up according to..."* Members are asked to line up according to various criteria, such as height or age, and they respond by creating a line that covers the continuum from one extreme to the other.

4. *Blind clap.* Members are asked to stand in a circle facing out so they cannot see each other. They are asked to clap their hands whenever they are so inclined and see if they can end up all clapping together, slowly, in the same rhythm.

5. *Paired challenge.* Members pair and decide who is A and B. Instructions are given such as: "As, count backward from 30 in 3s. Bs, name an animal and a plant that begin with the letter "e," etc.

6. *Dance challenge.* Teach group members a complicated contra dance, line dance or folk dance sequence.

7. *Human knot.* Members stand in a cluster facing each other and reach out and grasp hands with two different people. Then the group tries to untie the human knot without disconnecting hands or hurting anyone. This can also be played with one member (a volunteer, perhaps the one most in need of cool-down, such as the most recent protagonist of a drama) functioning as the knot analyst, who stays outside the tangle and then instructs members how to move, one at a time, to untangle the knot.

8. *The way home.* Members are asked to describe, in detail, the route they take to get home. This can be done in pairs to save time.

9. *"I'm looking forward to..."* Members are asked to relate some things they are looking forward to in the coming week.

10. *Animal connections.* Members are asked to think of a different animal for each letter of their first name.

De-roling procedures

Any time a group member plays a role in a psychodrama or sociodrama, it is important to make sure the member has let go of that role as well as to ensure that other group members are no longer seeing him or her in the role. De-roling is, therefore, a public process. Here are some examples of ways to de-role.

1. *Stepping out of role and into your name.* The member can take a large step forward and state, "I am no longer Gillian's brother. I am Martin."

2. *Three differences.* The person, the member for whom they played a role, or group members can name three ways that this role player is different from the role played.

3. *Three adjectives.* The person, the member for whom they played a role, or group members can name three adjectives that describe the member as himself or herself.

4. *Unzipping the role.* The person imagines they are wearing the role like a garment and they mime unzipping it along all edges, removing it, putting it on a hanger, and hanging it up.

5. *Shaking off the role.* The member stretches and shakes until they feel the role has completely left their body, adding sound if they would like.

6. *Peeling off the role.* The member imagines that they are wearing the role like a second skin, and mimes peeling it off and tossing it in the rubbish.

7. *Choral recitation.* The group joins in a choral recitation of the member's full name as they step forward out of role and into self.

8. *Object placement.* If there was an object or scarf used with the role, the member may say, "I leave the role of Gordon's mother with this scarf," as they hand the scarf to a leader. The leader can then shake the role out of the scarf, away from the members, and return the scarf to being a scarf.

9. *The de-roling gate.* Members can create a gate or portal of de-roling. The member who was in role steps "through" and she or he claims self back by saying his or her own name.

10. *The scarf wash.* Members can use scarves to "wash" roles off each other, or can stand in a double line, like a car wash, and have those who need to be de-roled pass between the washing scarves.

References

Blatner, A. (1996) *Acting In: Practical Applications of Psychodramatic Methods in Everyday Life*, 3rd edn. New York: Springer.

Blatner, A. (2000) *Foundations of Psychodrama: History, Theory, and Practice*, 4th edn. New York: Springer.

Clayton, G.M. (1994) *Effective Group Leadership*. Caulfield, Victoria: ICA Press.

Cossa, M. (2002) 'Drago-Drama: Archetypal sociodrama with adolescents.' In A. Bannister and A. Huntington (eds) *Communicating with Children and Adolescents: Action for Change.* London: Jessica Kingsley Publishers, pp.139–152.

Cossa, M. (2003) 'Taming puberty: Utilizing psychodrama, sociodrama, and sociometry with adolescent groups.' In J. Gershoni (ed.) *Psychodrama in the 21st century: Clinical and Educational Applications.* New York: Springer, pp.135–150.

Cossa, M., Ember, S., Glass, L. and Hazelwood, J. (1996) *ACTING OUT: The Workbook – A Guide to the Development and Presentation of Issue-Oriented, Audience-Interactive, Improvisational Theatre.* Muncie, IN: Accelerated Development/Bristol, PA: Taylor & Francis.

Emunah, R. (1990) 'Expression and expansion in adolescence: The significance of creative arts therapy.' *The Arts in Psychotherapy 17*, 101–107.

Erikson, E.H. (1950) *Childhood and Society*. New York: Norton.

Gordon, R. (2001) *What Should Happen in Adolescent Groups: Decoding and Directing the Chaos of Adolescent Group Life.* Melbourne: Fifth Pacific Rim Congress of IAGP.

Holmes, P. and Karp, M. (eds) (1991) *Psychodrama: Inspiration and Technique.* New York: Tavistock/Routledge.

Hudgins, M.K. (2002) *Treating PTSD in Action: The Therapeutic Spiral.* New York: Springer.

Jackins, H. (1966) *The Human Side of Human Beings: The Theory of Re-evaluation Counseling.* Seattle: Rational Island.

Kellermann, P.F. (1990) *Focus on Psychodrama: The Therapeutic Aspects of Psychodrama.* London: Jessica Kingsley Publishers.

Kellermann, P.F. and Hudgins, M.K. (eds) (2000) *Psychodrama with Trauma Survivors: Acting Out your Pain.* London: Jessica Kingsley Publishers.

Kübler-Ross, E. (1971) 'The five stages of dying.' *Encyclopedia Science Supplement.* New York: Grolier, pp.92–97.

Langs, R. (1981) *Psychotherapy: A Basic Text.* New York: Aronson.

Leveton, E. (2001) *A Clinician's Guide to Psychodrama*, 3rd edn. New York: Springer, pp.109–120.

Mahler, M.S., Pine, F. and Bergman, A. (1975) *The Psychological Birth of the Human Infant.* London: Hutchinson.

Miller, J.B. (1986) *Toward a New Psychology of Women.* Boston: Beacon Press.

Moreno, J.L. (1941) *The Words of the Father.* Beacon, NY: Beacon House.

Moreno, J.L. (1944) *The Theatre of Spontaneity.* Beacon, NY: Beacon House.

Moreno, J.L. (1959) *Psychodrama, Second Volume* Beacon, NY: Beacon House.

Moreno, J.L. (1964) *Psychodrama, First Volume* 3rd edn. Beacon, NY: Beacon House.

Moreno, J.L. (1993) *Who Shall Survive?* Roanoke, VA: Royal.

Moreno, J.L. (1994) 'Psychodrama moral philosophy and ethics.' In P. Holmes, M. Karp and M. Watson (eds) *Psychodrama since Moreno: Innovations in Theory and Practice.* London: Routledge, pp.97–111.

Moreno, J.L. and Moreno, Z. (1975) *Psychodrama, Third Volume* 6th edn. Beacon, NY: Beacon House.

National Association for Drama Therapy (2005) *www.nadt.org*

Piaget, J. (1963) *Origins of Intelligence in Children.* New York: Norton.

Resnick, M.D., Bearman, P.S., Blum, R.W., Bauman, K.E., Harris, K.M., Jones, J., Tabor, J., Beuhring, T., Sieving, R.E., Shew, M., Ireland, M., Bearinger, L.H. and Udry, J.R. (1997) 'Protecting adolescents from harm: Findings from the National Longitudinal Study on Adolescent Health.' *Journal of the American Medical Association 278,* 823–832.

Robson, M. (2000) 'Psychodrama with adolescent sexual offenders.' In P.F. Kellermann and M.K. Hudgins (eds) *Psychodrama with Trauma Survivors: Acting out your Pain.* London: Jessica Kingsley Publishers, pp.117–155.

Rohnke, K. (1989) *Cowtails and Cobras II: A Guide to Games, Initiatives, Ropes Courses, and Adventure Curriculum.* Debuque: Kendall/Hunt.

Rustin, T. and Olsson, P. (1993) 'Sobriety shop – a variation on magic shop for addiction treatment patients.' *Journal of Group Psychotherapy, Psychodrama and Sociometry 46,* 1, 12–23.

Sternberg, P. and Garcia, A. (1994) *Sociodrama: Who's in your Shoes?* Westport, CT: Praegar.

Therapeutic Spiral International (2005) *www.therapeuticspiral.org*

Tuckman, B.W. and Jensen, M.A.C. (1977) 'Stages of small group development revisited.' *Group and Organizational Studies 2,* 4, 419–427.

Winnicott, D.W. (1958) *Maturational Processes and the Facilitating Environment.* New York: International Universities Press.

Yalom, I.D. (1995) *Theories and Practice of Group Psychotherapy.* New York: Basic Books.

Subject Index

ability
  fluctuation within groups
    167
  working with differing
    145–6
absences
  notifying leaders 71
  rehearsing 126–9
abuse, within groups 67,
  68–9
abusive relationships, action
  techniques 116, 144–5
acceptance, termination stage
  40
accountability 50
*ACTING OUT: The Workbook
  – A Guide to the Development
  and Presentation of Issue-oriented, Audience-interactive,
  Improvisational Theatre*
  (Cossa *et al.*) 18, 90, 157
ACTINGOUT 18, 40–1, 67,
  75, 77–8, 127–8, 132
action, developing norms for
  stopping 154–5
action groups *see* adolescent
  groups
action locogram 113–14
action spectrogram 112–13
action techniques
  beginning stage 77–90
    initial contact with
      group members
      77–81
    introductory group
      sessions 81–5
    developing 85–90
  defined 22
  expression of feelings 48
  special populations
    138–52
  special settings/situations
    152–8
  suitability for adolescent
    groups 24–6
  termination stage
    123–33
    awareness of ending
      124–5
    rehearsals for
      ending 125–30
    process of termina-
      tion 130–3

therapeutic opportunity
  33
transition stage 91–9
  getting unstuck
    91–7
  moving forward
    97–9
working stage 101–21
  building strengths
    102–5
  developing observ-
    ing ego 105–8
  containment of
    intense affect
    108–12
  working with life
    issues 112–20
actual reality 29–30, 125
ADD/ADHD *see* attention
  deficit/hyperactivity
  disorder
adolescence 35–51
  defined 24
  developmental continuum
    emotional develop-
      ment 46–8
    mental development
      45–6
    personal develop-
      ment 48–50
    physical develop-
      ment 43–4
    social development
      50–1
  developmental tasks
    interpersonal 42
    personal 41–2
    transpersonal 42–3
  group development
    beginning stage
      36–7
    termination stage
      40–1
    transition stage
      37–9
    working stage
      39–40
  intensity of 25, 46
  therapeutic opportunity
    21–2
  see also young people
adolescent groups
  containment of intense
    affect 109, 111–12
  development *see* group/
    individual develop-
    ment

practical considerations
  159–68
  fitting strategies to
    actual needs
    162–7
  integrating theory
    and philosophy
    159–62
suitability of action
  methods 24–6
therapeutic opportunity
  21–2
therapeutic spiral 53–61
  containment 58–61
  observation 57–8
  restoration 54–6
adults, importance in adolescent development 42
affect
  dealing productively with
    58–61
  fluctuation with groups
    167
  working with intense
    108–12
Alliteration Circle 82–3
ambivalence, concretizing
  115, 191
amygdala 46
anger, termination stage 40
animal connections 195
animal movements 190–1
anorexia, working with 148
anti-social young people,
  working with 143–4
archetypal drama 105,
  119–20
art, as metaphor 93
artwork, building strengths
  105
"As I leave the group, I am
  taking with me…" 194
attention deficit/hyperactivity
  disorder, working with
  138–40
Autonomy vs. Shame and
  Doubt 38

baggage claim 192
balancing bodies 190
bargaining, termination stage
  40
beginning stage
  action techniques 77–90
    initial contact with
      group members
      77–81

beginning stage *cont.*
    introductory group
      sessions 81–5
      developing 85–90
  awareness of ending
    124–5
  group development
    36–7
behaviour, experimenting with
  25, 48
best friends 50
blind clap 195
Body Double 60, 61,
  109–12
bound/free movement 188
boundaries, working with
  85–8
brain development 43, 44,
  45, 46, 58, 60
building a group structure
  187

Canon of Creativity 160
central concerns, exploring
  114
chain improvisations, about
  endings 194
challenge by choice 70
challenge games 166
changing perspectives 106–7
chaos, moving away from
  97–9
Chaos Riders 97
childhood trauma victims,
  action techniques 144–5
Children's Performing Arts
  Center (CPAC) 17
children's stories, enacting
  193
choice, participation 70
choral recitation 196
circle of safety 102
Circle of Scarves 102–3
Circle of Similarities 83–4
client role 57
Closing Circles 80, 181–6
closing rituals 102–3
closure, unexpected departures
  130
co-leading/team leading
  64–6
coaching 60
collage, building strengths
  105
collage of my life 191
collective story telling 188

community norms, working
  within 162
competence
  building for psychodrama
    115
  group leader's role in
    building 153
  issues, emotional devel-
    opment 48
concretizing
  ambivalence 115, 191
  negative roles 153–4
confidence, leaders' role in
  building 153
confidentiality 67–8, 170,
  177
Conforti, Michael 63–4
containers, leaders' requirement to provide 73
Containing Double 60,
  109–12
containment 43
  of intense affect 108–12
  role of 58–61
  within groups 164–5
  young people with
    ADD/ADHD 139
cool-downs 118, 194–5
corrective emotional experiences 36, 38, 39
cosmos, as therapeutic concept
  32–3
Cossa/Conforti Colander
  Corollary for Clinical
  Containment 63–4
counseling, in-school 157–8
countertransference,
  group-work-inspired
  64–5
counting to ten as a group
  187
cultural diversity, working
  with 148–50
cultural norms, respecting
  149

dance challenge 195
dance/movement therapy
  (DMT) 22
dating behaviors, group members 71–2
de-roling 118, 194–5
  after exploring problem
    of substance abuse
    147
  procedures 195–7
defense mechanisms 59–60

defensiveness, transition stage
  37–8
denial, termination stage 40
desert island sociodrama 192
developmental continuum
  emotional development
    46–8
  mental development
    45–6
  personal development
    48–50
  physical development
    43–4
  social development
    50–1
developmental tasks
  awareness of defensive
    structures 59
  interpersonal 42
  personal 41–2
  transpersonal 42–3
differentiation 37
differing ability, working with
  145–6
directors 23–4, 64
disclosure 70
disengagement 57–8
distancing 27
"doodah" management 65
doubles
  in psychodrama 60
  see also Body Double;
    Containment Double
Drago-Drama 105, 120
drama, ADD as subject for
  139
drama therapy
  defined 23–4
  exploring personal issues
    88–90
  see also psycho/socio/
    drama therapy
dramatic enactment *see* role
  play

early adolescence
  emotional development
    46–7
  mental development 45
  personal development
    49
  physical development
    43–4
  social development 50
eating disorders, working with
  147–8

educational/skills building groups 157
Effective Group Leadership (Clayton) 91
ego psychology 35
egocentricity 57
emotional development 46–8
emotional maturity 48
empathy 50
enactment *see* role play
endings *see* termination
energy, fluctuation with groups 167
engagement 57–8
expansive activities 164
expression of feelings
    experimentation with 48
    leaves of absence 128
extremes, exploration of 25
eye contact, boundary exploration 86
Eye Contact – Switch Places 79

fairy tales, enacting 193
families, sample information pack for 169–172
family contact 170
family portraits 190
family relationship progression sculptures 193
feedback, at termination 131
feedback posters 193–4
feeling cards 191
Formal Operations 41–2
friendship sculptures 193
friendships
    between group members 72
    mid-adolescence 50
frontal cortex 43, 45
full sharing 118
functional present 28
future projections 124–5, 129

gate, de-roling 196
gender biased expectations, development 38
gender fishbowl 193
general mills 189
getting unstuck 91–7, 165
gift and the mirror 193
good-enough group leaders 39, 64
good-enough parents 39, 64

graphic arts 165
grief, at termination stage 40, 123, 132–3
ground rules 66
group closure 118
group cohesion 39
group development *see* group/individual development
group discussions, confidentiality 67
group dynamics, exploring 114–15
Group Juggle 82, 166
group leaders
    confidentiality 67–8
    frustration during transition stage 99
    functions in psychodrama 64
    good-enough 39, 64
    leaves of absence, rehearsing 127–9
    provision of container 73
    role of 63–6
    single 152–5
    supporting personal development 49
group members
    action techniques
        to support suicidal members 142–3
        working with reactions to suicide 140–2
    initial contact with 77–81
    leaves of absence, rehearsing 126–7
    physical contact between 69
    relationships between 71–2, 180
group membership
    fluctuating 155–6
    working with changing 163–4
group norms
    ADD/ADHD 138–9
    agreeing at introductory sessions 81
    consistent enforcement of 144
    developing for stopping action 154–5
    importance of 66–73
    reviewing and discussing 37, 84–5, 96

sample 177–9
group sculpture 94, 103, 129
group sessions
    introductory 81–5
    maintaining shifting focus in 154
group structure, building 187
group-generated norms 84
group/individual development 35–41
    beginning stage 36–7
    overlap between stages 37
    termination stage 40–1
    transition stage 37–9
    working stage 39–40

herd mentality 50, 54
histrionia normalis 25
human knot 195

identity, with peer groups 50
Identity vs. Role Confusion (Erikson) 101
illegal substances
    forbidden with groups 69–70
    see also substance abuse
"I'm looking forward to…" 195
imagination, creating templates of success 124–5
in-school groups 156–8
incremental goals, setting 125
individual development
    parallels with group development 35–41
    working with 163–7
information pack, sample 169–172
information sessions 77–81
informed consent 78
infra-reality 29
Initiative vs. Guilt 39
inner critic 107
inner evaluator 107
inner space 28
inpatient facilities 156
insight, from parents and schools 170–1
intake forms 173–5
intake process 171
intense affect, working with 108–12
intensity of adolescence 25, 46

intensity of the moment 27
internal roles 53
interpersonal developmental
    tasks 36–7, 42
interpersonal psychodrama
    116–17
interpersonal relationships 54
interpersonal skills, benefits of
    practicing 25
interpersonal strengths
        building 102–5
        connecting to 54–5
intrapersonal, emergence of
    37
intrapsychic psychodrama 28,
    115–16
intrapsychic sociodrama 142
introductory group sessions
    81–5
invisible friend 193
isolation, feelings of 47
issue/words improvisation
    189

Kid/Parent Circle 79–80

language choices, within
    groups 69
late adolescence
    emotional development
        47
    mental development 45
    personal development
        49
    physical development 44
    social development 50
leader dependent nature,
    beginning stage 36
leadership see group leaders
leaves of absence, rehearsing
    126–9
life issues, working with
    112–20
"line up according to…" 195
listening to the silence 188
Live Action Role Players
    (LARPers) 120
locked facilities 156

Magic Shop 126, 147
Manager of Defenses 59–60,
    108–9
Manager of Healthy Function-
    ing 59
Mario Stick 128

mask-making series 193
meaning making 42
megalomania normalis 25
mental development 45–6
mid-adolescence
    emotional development
        47
    mental development 45
    personal development
        49
    physical development 44
    social development 50
midbrain 43, 45, 46, 58
minority groups, working
    with 150–1
mirror position 107
mirroring activity 190
movement, activities 97, 165,
    188, 190, 192, 194
movement of opposite quali-
    ties 190
moving forward 97–9
multiple activities 166

name games 82–3
naming and celebrating 92
negative roles, concretizing
    153–4
neocortex 58
non-judgemental witness role
    58
non-mainstream groups,
    working with 150–1
nonclinical settings 158
nondirected improvisation,
    exploring personal issues
    88–9
nonlinear nature of groups,
    working with 163–7
norm violation vignettes 85
norming stage, group develop-
    ment 66
norms
    and guidelines for pro-
        grams 171
    see also community norms;
        cultural norms; group
        norms

object constancy 36, 39
object placement 196
object relations theory 35
objectivity 57–8
objects as self 192
observation 43
    ability for 41

role 57–8
observing ego 57–8
    developing 105–8, 117
Opening Circles
    boundary exploration 85
    getting unstuck 92
    ideas for 181–6
    information sessions 78
    introductory group ses-
        sions 81–2
opening rituals 102–3
opposites, movement to
    explore 190

paired challenge 195
paired and group mirrors 190
Paired Introductions 83
paired relationships, in groups
    72
parallel processes
    individual and group
        development 35–41
    leadership pairs and
        groups 64–5
parents
    communication with
        67–8
    good-enough 39, 64
    input from 170–1
    sample information pack
        for 169–172
participation 70–1, 180
pass the mask 187
past, exploration of 27
peeling off the role 196
peer groups
    identity with 50
    interaction through role
        play 24
    interpersonal develop-
        mental tasks 42
permission forms 173–5
personal development 48–50
personal developmental tasks
    41–2
personal issues, exploring
    88–90
personal material, confidenti-
    ality 67
personal strengths
    building 102–5
    connecting to 55–6
perspectives, changing 106–7
philosophy, integrating with
    practice 159–62
physical challenges, games
    with 166

physical contact, between group members 69
physical development 43–4
portal, de-roling 196
portal into the future 190
power continuum 191
practice, integrating theory and philosophy with 159–62
practicing stage 37
prescriptive roles 53, 54
  see also containment; observation; restoration
prevention curricula 24–5, 119
program norms 171
program participation 171
progression 163
progression sculptures, family relationship 193
props, non-directed improvisation 88–9
psycho/socio/drama therapy 119–20
  exploring problem of substance abuse 146–7
psychodrama
  building competence for 115
  building strengths 104
  cautions and complexities in 117–18
  defined 22–3
  differences between drama therapy and 23–4
  the double in 60
  eating disorders 147–8
  exploring problem of substance abuse 146
  functions of director/ group leader 23–4, 64
  potential to retraumatize 27
  sociodrama as training ground for 90
  to support suicidal group members 142–3
  warming up to holidays 125–6
  working with life issues 115–17
  working with reactions to suicide 141

  see also role play; role reversal; role training
Psychodrama in the 21st Century (Cossa) 91
Psychodrama since Moreno (Moreno) 32
Psychodrama, Third Volume (Moreno and Moreno) 26
psychotherapy
  thoughts on 169–170
  universalia of 19, 26–33
puberty 43–4
punctuality, as group norm 70–1

quadrant work 192

Rabbit/Tiger/Dragon 116
rapprochement 38
reality, as therapeutic concept 29–32
"rebel with a cause" roles 49
reclaiming roles 131–2
record keeping 172
reflection in movement 194
regression 163
rehearsals, for endings 125–30
relational therapy 38
relationships
  between group members 71–2, 180
  see also abusive relationships; friendships; interpersonal relationships
relationships through movement 192
religious observance issues, respecting 150
respect 68–70, 177–8
restoration, role of 54–6
retraumatization 27
rhythm circle 189
role awareness 107
role cards 191
role functions 53
role play 31–2
  building up energy in groups 166–7
  changing perspectives 106–7
  safe space 24, 25
role reversal 31
  activity demonstrating 80

building strengths 104
  with a character 188
  eating disorders 148
  with non-mainstream groups 151
  strengthening observing ego 107–8
role training 31
  supporting recovery from substance abuse 147
  working with life issues 119
roles
  "rebel with a cause" 49
  reclaiming at termination 131–2
  see also de-roling; negative roles; prescriptive roles
romantic involvement
  between group members 71
  societal pressures 46–7

safe space, action group as 24, 25, 48, 68
safety, internalized sense of 39
sample group norms 177–9
sample information pack 169–172
Santa's workshop 126
scarf circle 102–3
scarf wash 196
scene setting 28
scenes, highlights of groups 194
scenic psychodrama 117
school bus 189–90
school officials, communication with 67–8
schools, input from 170–2
scrapbooks 192
scripted material 120
scripted theatre 24
secrets, telling 192–3
Secure Frame Dread 38, 92
seek and point 195
selection process 171
self
  development of 48
  objects as 192
self-portraits, through collage 105
self-soothing 109
self-talk 60, 109
separation anxiety 40

separation/individuation 37, 38
Sex, Drugs and Rock & Roll 17
sexual activity 47
sexual development 46
sexual orientation 47
shaking off the role 196
sharing
 during boundary exploration 88
 during information sessions 80–1
 leadership role 153
shield of self-confidence 105
shifting focus, in group sessions 154
single group leaders 152–5
snapshots, highlights of groups 194
Sobriety Shop 147
social development 50–1
social roles, exploring 25
societal pressures, romantic involvement 46–7
Sociodrama: Who's in Your Shoes (Sternberg and Garcia) 115
sociodrama
 building strengths 104
 defined 22–3
 desert island 192
 exploring personal issues 89–90
 with non-mainstream groups 151
 to support suicidal group members 142
 transition stage 96–7
 warming up to holidays 125–6
 working with life issues 114–15
 working with reactions to suicide 141–2
 see also psycho/socio/drama therapy
sociometric activities
 introductory group sessions 83–4
 power of 94–5
 transition stage 94
 working with life issues 112–14
 working stage 103
Sociometric Map 80
sociometry, defined 23

space, as therapeutic concept 28–9
special populations, working with 138–52
special settings/situations, working in 152–8
spectrograms 84
spiritual dimension, in therapy 43
spontaneity 28, 160
stepping out of role and into your name 195
storming phase, group development 91
storytelling, collective 188
strength cards 104
strengths
 building 102–5
 connecting to 54–6
stress, within groups 164
Stretch band 189
substance abuse
 exploring the problem 146–7
 supporting recovery through role training 147
 see also illegal substances
suicidal thinking 140
suicidal young people, working with 140–3
supervision, in leadership 65–6
support groups, in-school 157–8
surplus reality 30–2, 119, 124, 125, 151
symbiotic stage 36–7

tag-word improvisation 187
team leading 64–6
teasing 68–9
"tell me about the time when…" 187–8
telling secrets 192–3
tense and relax 188
termination anxiety 40
termination issues 72–3, 180–1
termination stage
 action techniques 123–33
  awareness of endings 124–5
  rehearsals for endings 125–30

 process of termination 130–3
 group development 40–1
terminology 22–4
territoriality 28
testing behaviors 91
theatrical experience, working with young people with 151–2
theory, integrating with practice 159–62
Therapeutic Spiral Model™ (TSM) 53–61
 containment 58–61
 observation 57–8
 restoration 54–6
therapy, thoughts on 169–170
thinking
 early adolescence 45
 suicidal 140
three adjectives 196
three changes 188–9
Three Containers Exercise 87–8
three differences 196
time, in psychotherapy 26–8
time issues, psychodrama 118
time travel, to final meeting 124
timeline activities 130–1
TNO (That's Not OK) 69
touch blue 194–5
transference, group-work-inspired 64–5
transition stage
 action techniques 91–9
  getting unstuck 91–7
  moving forward 97–9
 group development 37–9
transpersonal, search for 33
transpersonal developmental tasks 42–3
transpersonal strengths
 building 102–5
 connecting to 56
trauma dramas 118
trauma victims
 non-judgmental development 58
 working with young 144–5
trust, leaders' role in building 153

Trust vs. Mistrust 36, 54
two scarves 193

unexpected departures,
    rehearsing 129–30
universalia of psychotherapy
    19, 26–33
unspoken norms 66
unzipping the role 196
upgrading, childhood chal-
    lenges 101

vignettes 96
VOTE, exploring personal
    issues 90

warm-up activities
    before holidays 125–6
    boundary exploration
        86–7
    dramatic 166
    exploring life issues 116
    ideas for 186–94
    information sessions 79
    working stage 103
the way home 195
westernization 149–50
"what I wish I had told you
    is…" 188
who started the movement?
    187
witness role, non-judgmental
    58
The Words of the Father
    (Moreno) 32
working stage
    action techniques
        101–21
        building strengths
            102–5
        containment of
            intense affect
            108–12
        developing observ-
            ing ego 105–8
        working with life
            issues 112–20
    group development
        39–40
worst day tableaux 191

young adults
    emotional development
        48
mental development
    45–6
personal development
    49–50
physical development 44
social development 51
young people
    action techniques
        ADD/ADHD
            138–40
        anti-social and
            sociopathic
            143–4
        childhood trauma
            victims 144–5
        with differing
            abilities 145–6
        eating disorders
            147–8
        from different
            cultures 148–50
        non-mainstream
            groups 150–1
        substance abuse
            146–7
        suicidal 140–3
        with theatre
            experience 151–2
    see also adolescence; ado-
        lescent groups
youth educators 25
youth prevention education
    24–5
Youth Services, Inc. (YSI) 17

Author Index

Blatner, A. 118

Clayton, G.M. 91
Cossa, M. 90, 91, 105, 120, 157

Emunah, R. 21, 164
Erikson, E.H. 35, 36, 38, 39, 54, 101

Garcia, A. 115
Gordon, R. 160

Holmes, P. 159
Hudgins, M.K. 19, 43, 51, 53, 60, 65, 75, 101, 102, 145

Jackins, H. 78
Jensen, M.A.C. 91

Karp, M. 159
Kellermann, P.F. 64, 145
Kübler-Ross, E. 40

Langs, R. 38, 92
Leveton, E. 126

Mahler, M.S. 35, 36, 37, 38, 39
Miller, J.B. 35, 38
Moreno, J.L. 19, 22, 23, 25, 26, 28, 29, 30, 31, 32, 33, 48, 101, 160
Moreno, Z. 19, 26, 28, 29, 31, 33

National Association for Drama Therapy 23

Olsson, P. 147

Piaget, J. 41

Resnick, M.D. 42
Rohnke, K. 70
Rustin, T. 147

Sternberg, P. 115

Therapeutic Spiral International 60
Tuckman, B.W. 91

Winnicott, D.W. 35, 39

Yalom, I.D. 38